NURSING ESSENTIALS MODULE

for NCLEX-RN
with Critical Thinking Exercises

Carol Bininger, RN, PhD
S. Kim Genovese, RNC, MSN, MSA
Kathleen M. Maher, RN, MSN
Kay Scharn, RN, MSN, EdS
Nancy Wallace, RN,C, MSN
James Lile, PharmD

STAFF

Clinical Editor
Marguerite S. Ambrose, RN,CS, MSN, CCRN

Clinical Reviewer
Judith E. Meissner, RN, MSN

Copy Editor
Jane Benner

Cover Design
Jake Smith

CONTRIBUTORS

Nursing Fundamentals
Kathleen M. Maher, RN, MSN

Mental Health Nursing
Carol Bininger, RN, PhD
Gail Iglesias, RN, EdD

Pediatric Nursing
Nancy Wallace, RN,C, MSN

Medical/Surgical Nursing
Kay Scharn, RN, MSN, EdS

Maternity Nursing
S. Kim Genovese, RNC, MSN, MSA

Pharmacology
James Lile, PharmD

CONTENTS

Ace It! Nursing Essentials Module

CHAPTER 5 - **Maternity nursing**

CHAPTER 6 - **Pediatric nursing**

CHAPTER 7 - Medical/surgical nursing

Chapter 8 - **Pharmacology review**

CHAPTER 1

Nursing Fundamentals

LEGAL ISSUES IN NURSING PRACTICE

State laws affecting nursing practice vary from state to state. Nurses are responsible for knowing the laws regulating the practice of nursing in their state. When practicing nursing in any setting, nurses should adhere to the following guidelines:

- Follow the standards of clinical nursing practice established by the American Nurses Association (ANA).
- Follow policies of employing organization as long as they do not conflict with state board regulations or ANA standards of practice.
- Seek consultation when in doubt about the protocol to use with any client.
- Document what you did and said; what the client did and said; who you consulted with; what you did as a result of any consultation with another; any changes in client behavior. Documentation is the nurse's best defense in the event of a lawsuit.

A. **Tort** (violation of a person's private rights)

   Torts are classified as unintentional (negligence) and intentional (assault and battery).

B. **Informed consent**
   1. Clients have a right to know about the prescribed treatments and to decide whether to participate.
   2. Clients cannot be forced to accept a treatment unless a court deems they are incompetent to make an informed decision (i.e., a client who is actively suicidal may be required to accept treatment until the suicidal crisis passes).
   3. Clients whose ability to reason is impaired (i.e., advanced Alzheimer's disease) will need to have a guardian appointed who can give informed consent.
   4. In most states, minors cannot give informed consent.
   5. Informed consent can be revoked by the client at any time.
   6. Failure to obtain informed consent can result in a lawsuit against all who provide treatment or care.

C. **Confinement**
   1. Clients who seek voluntary admission to a psychiatric facility have the right to be discharged at will within the guidelines of the facility and the state law.
   2. Clients admitted to a psychiatric facility against their will can be detained no longer than 72 hours without a court order.

D. Use of seclusion or restraints

1. Use of seclusion and/or restraints must fall within guidelines specified by state law and hospital policy.
2. The principle of least restrictive environment must be followed.
3. Accurate documentation of the behavior leading to restraint is required and imperative.
4. If the client is restrained or secluded, agency policies for care must be scrupulously followed.

E. Assault and battery

1. Assault is the attempt, or threat, to unlawfully touch or injure another person. Battery is the actual unlawful and intentional touching of another.
2. Nurses need to be aware of situations that are associated with assault and battery (i.e., involuntary commitment, invading the client's space, past history of poor impulse control).
3. Nurses need to know how to handle clients who need physical restraint to avoid harming the client.
4. Nurses should follow agency policy and procedure when intervening with clients who are out of control.

F. Client rights

1. Hospitalization does not deprive clients of due process.
2. Clients have the right to the least restrictive environment for treatment.
3. Although psychiatrists may have the right to privileged communication with their clients, nurses are generally not accorded the same privilege.
4. Exceptions to maintaining confidentiality can include a client reporting child abuse or intent to harm another. The nurse needs to follow state law and agency policy regarding exceptions to confidentiality.
5. Nurses cannot release information to third parties about the client without the client's written consent.

G. Documentation of care

1. Documentation of care is essential to protect a nurse in the event of a lawsuit.
2. Records must be accurate and objective (descriptive).
3. Any changes in client behaviors must be noted.
4. Refrain from using such phrases as "Client remains the same." or "No change in client's behavior." Describe what you observe.

5. Remember, if it is not documented, it did not happen! Courts rely on what is in the record, not what comes from memory.

THERAPEUTIC COMMUNICATION

Definition
The planned, deliberate verbal and non-verbal interaction between a caregiver (nurse) and a client that promotes a healing and assisting relationship.

Defining characteristics
1. Goal directed and purposeful
2. Increases person's ability to function and builds self-esteem
3. Promotes spiritual restoration
4. Verbal and nonverbal

Differences between social and therapeutic communication
1. Social communication
   a. Builds mutual pleasure
   b. Is noncontractual
   c. Is timeless
   d. Involves sharing and mutual giving and receiving
2. Therapeutic communication
   a. Is singularly focused on the client; the therapist gives and the client receives
   b. Requires a contract between the therapist and client
   c. Has a time limit
   d. Has a healing purpose
   e. Requires special understanding of behavior models

Techniques of therapeutic communication
1. Silence--not talking lets the client collect his thoughts and analyze his feelings
2. Self-disclosure--discussing information that is personal to the therapist helps convey understanding of what the client is saying
3. Suggestion--provides alternatives for the client to consider
4. Confrontation--challenges inconsistencies, untruths, and evasions
5. Concreteness--clarifies what the client is telling the therapist
6. Genuineness--honestly answers asked questions
7. Immediacy--recognizes what is happening between the therapist and the client as it happens
8. Empathy--feeling how the client feels temporarily

9. Respect--conveys a sincere desire to listen to what the client has to say without being judgmental
10. Reflection--paraphrasing what the client has just said
11. Restating--repeating what the client has just said to show that the therapist is listening
12. Focusing--helps the client view a subject more deeply

Actions that promote therapeutic communication
1. Assess client's behavior
2. Analyze the client's needs
3. Plan the therapeutic goals with the client
4. Act in ways that build self-esteem
5. Avoid conflicting roles
6. Evaluate outcomes

CHARACTERISTICS OF
SOCIAL AND THERAPEUTIC RELATIONSHIPS

In an effective nurse-client relationship, the nurse uses therapeutic communication to shed light on, provide insight, and develop positive changes in the client's behavior. This chart contrasts important differences between a therapeutic relationship and a social one.

Social relationship
- Focuses on mutual sharing, with each participant giving and receiving
- Promotes mutual pleasure
- Has no time constraints
- Does not involve a contract
- Does not require the participants to examine their behavior or possess a specialized knowledge base

Therapeutic relationship
- Focuses on the client, with the nurse giving and the client receiving
- Promotes client healing
- Is time-limited
- Involves a contract between nurse and client
- Requires the nurse to have a sound understanding of human behavior and to examine the nurse's and the client's behaviors from a theoretical perspective

GRIEVING

Overview

Grief and the act of grieving are universal and some of the most strongly felt emotional states. They influence all parts of a person's life, causing a wide range of psychological and physiological manifestations. The suffering may last a matter of days or continue for weeks or months.

Grief is the result of a loss. The loss of a loved one, a body part, a favorite object, a loved pet, or a job; being diagnosed with a serious illness; or having a change in life's status are examples of losses that may precipitate grief. The person experiencing grief becomes withdrawn and preoccupied with self.

Responses to grieving can be adaptive (uncomplicated) or maladaptive (pathologic). Adaptive grief is self-limiting and travels a relatively expected path (see "Adaptive grieving stages" below). Maladaptive grief is the suppression of an emotional response and may follow two courses: delayed reaction or distorted reaction. A person who experiences no emotion following a loss may be experiencing a delayed grief reaction. In many cases the delayed reaction manifests itself later, often on the anniversary of the loss. A distorted reaction to grief is clinical depression. It can be severe and incapacitating, requiring professional intervention.

Knowledge of the grieving process has important implications for nurses who face many situations with clients who are at risk for suffering a major loss. The importance of the lost person or object to the client needs to be assessed so proper responses may be made to help the client develop an adaptive response to the resulting grief.

ADAPTIVE GRIEVING STAGES

Persons who follow an adaptive response to a loss will pass through five constant stages. Stages are relative and may last for months and even years.

Stages	Clinical behaviors	Nursing interventions
1. Denial	Avoids talking about loss. Won't look at surgical wound. Ignores teachings. Withdraws from others.	Answer only what client asks. Explain all care being given. Provide emotional support to client and family. Listen to client--do not argue.
2. Anger	Becomes a complainer. Blames others for current predicament. The nurse often becomes focus of anger.	Speak in present tense as client is not ready for the future. Allow anger outbursts without comment.
3. Bargaining	Expresses desire to be a better person. If disease is cured, promises to change life style.	Speak realistically. Do not get drawn into client's bargaining. Teach in the present tense--client is not ready for the future.
4. Resolution	Emotional reality begins. Client realizes the reality of the loss and begins to question alternatives to deal with it.	Encourage emotional expressions. Provide information about the future. Be available at client's request.
5. Acceptance	The reality of the loss is accepted. Self-confidence returns and client begins to assert independence.	Focus on the future. Teach skills that may be needed to cope with the loss. Bring family into discussions. Teach about support groups, if appropriate.

CASE MANAGEMENT PRINCIPLES

Overview

Over the past decade there have been major additions to the system of health care delivery in the United States. These new alternatives have led to the proliferation of health maintenance organizations (HMOs), preferred provider organizations (PPOs), and managed care. The concept of managed care dominated the delivery of health care in the nineties and probably will do so well into the twenty-first century. With this domination, the distinctions between delivery systems (HMOs, PPOs) has become unclear, having in common only the features of pre-negotiated payment for services, pre-certification for care, utilization review, and limited choices in selecting a health-care provider. The concept of managed care has its roots in the public health nursing model, which provided for one nurse to assume responsibility for meeting (managing) a number of clients' and families' health care needs. The managed care delivery system has created the need for a specialized health delivery practitioner: the case manager. Professional nurses, by virtue of the breath of their education and experience, are ideal case managers.

A case management model

A. Definition and description

1. Case management is a systematic approach to delivering total client care within specified time frames and economic resources.
2. Case management includes the client's entire illness episode, crosses all care settings in which care is received, and involves collaborating with all health personnel who care for the client.
3. Case managers focus on coordinating care for a client group with complex health care requirements usually having similar diagnoses and needs and requiring common therapies.

B. Case management goals

1. To direct client care that is:
   - good quality
   - appropriate
   - timely
   - cost-effective
2. Case management goals remain the same regardless of the care setting.

C. Case management critical pathways

1. Critical pathways are guidelines that lay out interdisciplinary care

plans that must be carried out for a group of clients (case load).
2. Critical pathways are the tools for monitoring the case-load process to assure reaching the desired outcomes.
3. Critical pathways may be:
   - Medical--drug orders, diagnostic procedures, prescriptions for therapies.
   - Nursing--comfort interventions, client-teaching activities, self-care activities, all within the constraints of time and cost.
4. Critical pathways are followed regardless of the health care setting.

D. Case manager roles
1. Case managers are responsible for delivering appropriate health care in a timely and cost-effective manner.
2. They assure that critical pathways are designed and used to achieve desired client outcomes.
3. They refer clients to the multi-disciplinary care team.
4. They supervise discharge planning.
5. Case managers provide the client with the best resources to meet the care plan. They troubleshoot for the client if problems occur.
6. They use quality assurance programs to evaluate the quality, timeliness, and cost effectiveness of client care.

E. Characteristics of a case manager
1. According to guidelines established by the ANA, nurse case managers should:
   - Have a baccalaureate degree in nursing and a master's degree and be certified as a clinical nurse specialist in the client's disease area.
   - Have 3 years' clinical nursing experience.
2. They should possess the expert knowledge necessary to set client goals and outcomes; clearly understand and be willing to work within the financial constraints of current health care systems; be skilled at developing strategies for quality improvement.
3. Case managers must have highly developed skills of communication, negotiation, and collaboration with other health care providers.
4. They must know what resources are available in health care facilities and the client's community.

HOME HEALTH NURSING

Overview

The move of the American health care delivery system to managed care has accelerated the need for providing more health care in the home. Chronic health problems that used to receive periodic care in a hospital now are cared for exclusively at home. Early discharge of clients who have had surgery or an acute illness episode has raised the acuity level of clients in home care. The increase in the elderly population who have more chronic illnesses being treated at home has raised the level of skills required by the caregivers. Nurses, the traditional providers of community-based care, are being called upon by the federal government, through Medicare regulations, home health agencies, and insurance providers, to direct the delivery of home health nursing, both skilled and unskilled. The effective providing of home health nursing requires enhanced clinical skills and an understanding of rules and regulations of home care.

Home health care services

1. Home health care delivers multi-disciplinary health services to clients and their families where they live.
2. The goal of home health care is to restore an optimum functional level for the client and foster family independence.
3. Home health nursing services include:
   - Skilled nursing care.
   - Teaching health care.
   - Collaborating among all professional health-care providers to assure cooperation, continuity of care, and compliance with government eligibility requirements.
   - Identifying and communicating to the client and family the community resources that can help achieve the care plan outcomes.
4. Ancillary home health service providers
   - Home health aides
   - Housekeepers
   - Companions
5. Home health care equipment
   - Beds and ambulatory aids
   - Portable dialysis units
   - Ventilators and infusion pumps

Factors that influence effective home nursing
1. Educating the family about the problem for which care is being given.
2. Using educated professionals with the relevant skills to deal with the health problem.
3. Establishing effective social support services.
4. Maintaining appropriate living environment.
5. Developing reliable transportation and locating a local emergency health facility.
6. Having competent care managers.

Home health nurses' responsibilities
1. Clinical responsibilities
   - Wound care--debriding and irrigating wounds; assessing wound healing; teaching wound care.
   - Drug therapy compliance--teaching drug actions, drug adverse effects and administration schedules; monitoring drug therapy effectiveness and client compliance.
   - Nutrition--assessing client's nutritional status; administering tube and parenteral feedings; teaching good nutrition habits; monitoring diet compliance.
   - Elimination--providing enterostomal care; teaching client and family use of irrigation catheters and good skin care; monitoring client for infection.
   - Mobility--demonstrating use of assistive devices; performing range-of-motion exercises.
   - Infection control--teaching family universal precautions; monitoring home environment for potential areas that promote infection.
2. Psychosocial responsibilities
   - Evaluating the client and family--socioeconomic factors in the home; cultural and family dynamics.
   - Recognizing that the home health nurse is a guest in the client's home.
   - Being non-judgmental about the client's beliefs.
   - Accepting the client's ability and willingness to learn.
3. Legal and ethical responsibilities
   - Complying with the laws and regulations regarding home care.
   - Working within an approved care plan.
   - Assuring that health care provider has collaborated on the treatment plan has been obtained.

- Assuring that written permission from the client or family to enter the home has been obtained.
- Maintaining confidentiality about the client's condition and treatment when asked by neighbors or family friends who may be present in the home.
- Providing documentation of care to assure continued and optimum reimbursement for the client.
- Understanding when and how to withdraw services when reimbursement authorization expires.

Assuring personal safety precautions
1. Know the neighborhood and the safest route into and out of it.
2. Carry agency, police, and emergency facility phone numbers.
3. Inform agency of daily visit schedule with each client's phone number.
4. Report in to agency by phone after each visit.
5. Do not drive an expensive automobile, wear expensive jewelry, or show a lot of money.
6. Do not enter the client's home if anyone there is intoxicated, hostile, or demonstrating obnoxious behavior.
7. Never enter a home unless invited. Promptly leave if you feel unsafe.

LEADERSHIP, MANAGEMENT, AND DELEGATION

Overview
The responsibilities of leadership, managing staff, and delegating client care responsibilities are inherent in all nursing positions. The process of leading, managing, and delegating is an interpersonal process requiring strong communication and interpersonal skills to effectively create change in others. To practice competently in today's health care climate, a professional nurse must be able to manage a variety of ancillary nursing personnel and appropriately delegate tasks that can legally be delegated.

Leadership and management, while similar, are not exactly the same. *Leadership* is the ability to influence the activities of others to achieve goals. *Management* is a form of leadership that focuses on achieving organizational goals. As a beginning nurse, you must be able to use the basic principles of leadership and management as you work with other nursing personnel to provide care for clients.

The primary functions of leadership include:
- *communicating*, both formally and informally, to members of a group
- *motivating* members of a group to behave in ways that achieve goals
- *initiating*, bringing something new, such as a nursing procedure, into the practice of a group
- **facilitating** the accomplishment of a task, considering the needs and group's goals
- *integrating*, bringing all the parts together.

The primary functions of management include:
- *planning*, mapping out beforehand how something will be achieved
- *organizing*, establishing a structure through which the plans are carried out
- *staffing*, hiring and scheduling staff in appropriate positions to carry out the plans
- *directing*, giving instructions and delegating tasks to staff members
- *controlling*, measuring the staff's performance by comparing it to established standards.

There are three basic leadership and management styles. No one style is appropriate in all situations. The *authoritarian* style is characterized by structure, order, and much more emphasis on accomplishing a task than on the people performing the task. This style is useful in crisis situations, such as codes or disasters. A *laissez-faire* or *permissive* style is characterized by little (if any) direction or control and may be useful when the group being lead is a highly motivated professional group, such as a research team. The *democratic* style of management focuses on collaboration and participation in decision making. It is useful in most work situations, because people usually work more effectively when they are part of the decision-making process.

Roles are how people are expected to act according to the societal position they hold. For example, a nursing instructor has a different role than a nursing student. Each person filling a role has expectations about what behaviors are expected in that role. In addition, other people, workplace standards, and society in general, all have expectations (very often different!) about how anyone in a certain role should behave. To further complicate matters, each of us fills more than one role. For example, a nursing instructor taking courses for an advanced degree is also a student. She may also be a wife, a mother, a daughter, and a sister.

When a person feels the need to conform to conflicting expectations, she'll experience *role conflict.* How she resolves that conflict can have either positive or negative effects on the social system and the individuals who are part of that system. When people in various positions in a group are dissatisfied, angry, or stressed, you as the leader can help analyze the roles of the people involved by asking several questions:
- What is the source of the conflict?
- Are the roles for the positions clearly defined?
- Do members of the group have different expectations for one or more of the roles?

Once you have analyzed the role conflict, there are several strategies that you can use to resolve the conflict.
- Ask the group members how they would describe the expectations of each role.
- Clarify any unclear role expectations, giving specific, clear explanations.
- If having too many demands is part of the problem, help each person set priorities.
- Identify ways in which individuals can diffuse anger or relieve stress.

You can use these strategies to resolve conflicts, whether you're dealing with one individual or with a group (for example, having a team conference). As you can see, communication skills are essential to being a competent leader.

Communication has two forms, interpersonal and organizational. *Interpersonal communication* is the process of passing a message from one person to another or to a small group. *Organizational communication* is the system used within an organization to communicate with its members. It may be *formal,* such as directives, newsletters, or group conferences, or *informal,* occurring established channels (often called the grapevine).

Communication flows in many directions in an organization, up from the staff to management, down from management to staff, and horizontally among people on the same organizational level. In nursing, there are special considerations associated with communication.

- Clients may share confidential information with their caregiver and have the right to expect that only *necessary* information will be shared with other caregivers.
- The change of shift report is an opportunity for an effective exchange of information to improve client care.
- Documenting the care given in the client's record validates that the care was indeed delivered, communicates vital information to other caregivers, and creates a permanent record.

Delegation

Another skill necessary to being a competent leader is working with groups. Developing group skills means learning to know and accept group members, agreeing on the group's purpose, and establishing a structure and process for accomplishing the group's goals. Group effectiveness is based on some fundamental essentials, including:

- clearly defined, measurable goals that the group has agreed upon and that conform to the organization's goals
- clearly defined expectations that are compatible with organization's expectations.

Serving in the RN's leadership role, you will be expected to carry out certain management activities. One of the most important and frequent of these is *delegating* tasks to others. Delegating tasks can help reduce health care costs by using your time more efficiently. Delegating will improve your performance by giving you time to focus on higher priorities, such as assigning a nursing assistant to feed a client so that you can assess a newly admitted client or provide discharge teaching. Delegating also helps workers gain confidence in their ability to perform and builds cooperation and team spirit.

The authority to delegate is based on law and regulation, so you must adhere to your state's standards for delegation to protect your nursing license. You can find these standards in your state's nurse practice act. While reviewing it keep the following questions in mind:

- Is delegation permitted?
- How is delegation defined?
- Who has the authority to delegate?
- Is the unlicensed assistive personnel's (UAP's) role defined?
- Does it authorize delegation based on circumstances?

- Are there any tasks that you cannot delegate?
- Does the nurse practice act indicate the consequences of inappropriate delegation?

Accountability

The question of accountability arises when discussing delegation. In the context of delegation, accountability means bearing responsibility for both the action and inaction of yourself and those to whom you delegate tasks. This means that you are accountable for all care-related nursing decisions. You are responsible to ensure appropriate assessment, planning, implementation, supervision, and evaluation. Only implementation of tasks can be delegated to UAPs.

To make the right decisions when delegating, you need to develop a relationship with any UAP working with you. Effective delegation depends on mutual trust. Be sure the UAP is comfortable enough with you to admit that she does not know how to do a task rather than doing something she is nor prepared to carry out. Also make sure that she understands that someone else can't do the task she has been assigned.

Legally, if you do not delegate appropriately or the UAP does a task that you have not authorized, you both are subject to legal action. While this may make you hesitate to delegate tasks, remember, appropriate delegation occurs when you understand the principles of delegation and implement them correctly. Your employer is also accountable and cannot mandate you to delegate nursing duties to UAPs.

The National Council of State Boards of Nursing (NCSBN) has outlined the five rights of delegation you can apply to your practice. They are:

Right task	Delegated tasks must conform to the established guidelines for UAPs. You must assess every client situation before delegating. Consider the client's condition, the UAP's capabilities, the complexity of the task, and how much supervision the UAP will require.
Right circumstances	You can delegate only implementation *tasks* because they do not require independent judgment.
Right person	You need to know that the UAP working with you has competency in certain tasks. Has she demonstrated this by completing the institution-required orientation program?
Right direction and communication	You need to communicate clearly about each delegated task. Provide specific information about what the UAP should report to you and when to report back. Be sure she understands your expectations.
Right supervision and evaluation	Assigning a task is not all that is involved in delegation. You also need to guide and supervise the UAP and evaluate the work being done to be sure that it meets your expectations. You should provide feedback and invite the UAP's feedback so you can assess the delegation process.

Delegating tips
• give clear, specific instructions, including objectives and expected results
• be familiar with the task, and anticipate possible problems and solutions
• be available to provide guidance and/or help if needed
• if possible, give the UAP some latitude as to how to complete the task
• provide feedback--positive reinforcement for a job well done or constructive comments indicating specific behaviors that need improvement if the task wasn't done as expected
• remember that, although a task may be delegated, the *responsibility* remains with you, the RN
• instill confidence; be patient, especially if the task is a new one

Prioritization

You are very familiar with determining priorities of care for individual clients. Many of the questions you will review as part of this course will test your ability to do this. As an RN, you will be expected to prioritize not only for individual clients, but also for groups of clients. To be successful, you will need to analyze the data available about all the clients, determine if any additional data are necessary, and make judgments about how to order the priorities. Each client care situation will have its own priorities, and no course or book could possibly address every conceivable situation. When answering NCLEX questions about prioritizing care, however, consider the following:

1. Safety needs supersede everything. For example, you would attend to a client in danger of lacerating himself with a sharp instrument before caring for a client complaining of chest pain.

2. Remember the ABCs (airway, breathing, and circulation). For example, a client with an arterial bleed takes precedence over one who is complaining of pain.

3. According to the nursing process, you must assess a client first before performing an intervention.

CHAPTER 2

PHYSICAL ASSESSMENT

Overview
Physical assessment is a systematic and organized process for collecting data about a client's health state. It is done on a regular schedule to maintain wellness and as necessary when a client complains of a health problem.

The physical assessment must be accurate, comprehensive, and thorough to produce sufficient data to make appropriate nursing diagnoses. The assessment should be holistic, exploring all bio-psychosocial factors of a client's life. All findings from the assessment should be documented following a prescribed organized format that is known and understood by all caregivers.

General principles for a physical assessment
1. Record gathered information as it is obtained to avoid omissions and inaccurate facts.
2. Organize the data systematically: subjective information first, objective information second.
3. Use clear appropriate language that is understandable. Use only common abbreviations.
4. Remember the record is a legal document. All facts should be stated objectively.
5. Inform the client about the data collecting. Respect the client's privacy and confidentiality.
6. Quantify any measurements and describe abnormalities in detail.

A complete physical assessment comprises three components: health history, physical examination, and laboratory diagnostic studies.

The health history
The health history is subjective information reported by the client in a personal interview. It is the client's view of his current health state. The health history should reveal:
1. Any health problems from his perspective.
2. Past medical history from childhood to present age.
3. Family history, including health of all close relatives, living and causes of death of those dead.
4. A personal profile of the client's social life, emotional well-being, sexuality, stress level, coping techniques, and use of substances.

The physical examination

The physical examination is the technique to collect objective information about the client's body. It may elicit information the client has not reported during the history taking and confirm what he described in the history interview. A physical examination begins when the examiner first sees the client and gets an initial impression of his demeanor, look, posture, facial and body expressions. The examination that follows evaluates all body systems' function and consists of using inspection, percussion, palpation, and auscultation to gather information.

Laboratory diagnostic studies

Diagnostic studies are an important source of information about a client's health. In many cases, these studies reveal important information that is not apparent in the history and physical examination. The client needs to have detailed teaching about diagnostics that will be done as part of the physical assessment. A description of the test and client preparation prior to it is essential for test accuracy and client comfort. Diagnostic study results should be analyzed in connection with the health history and physical examination. Results should be reviewed with the client.

COMMON DIAGNOSTIC TESTS

Introduction

This chapter describes 23 diagnostic tests and procedures that may appear on the NCLEX-RN. Each test is categorized by type (blood, urine, stool, x-ray, etc.) and listed alphabetically within the category. Some common tests are not covered here because they are covered in other *Ace It!* Modules. (An example is electrolytes, which are discussed in the Video Module.)

The normal values given for each test are relative. Normal ranges vary among health facilities. Therefore, you should always rely on the normal values accepted by your practice setting. The NCLEX-RN will reference generally accepted ranges. Test questions containing variations from normal will be so different from normal that you will recognize them as abnormal.

Blood tests

Test: AIDS serology

The enzyme-linked immunosorbent assay (ELISA) tests for a human immunodeficiency virus (HIV) antibodies in blood serum and plasma. It is the most sensitive and accurate validator of the presence of HIV antibodies.

- Normal values: No presence of HIV antibodies
- Conditions affecting test results: Leukemia, lymphoma, syphilis, and alcoholism may cause false-positive findings.
- Special nursing considerations:
    1. Be nonjudgmental when counseling clients about the test.
    2. Respect the client's wish for anonymity.
    3. Teach the client that the test does not mean that he has AIDS, but only that he has been exposed to the virus.
    4. Review safer-sex practices regardless of the test outcome.

Test: Bleeding time

Bleeding time evaluates platelet and microvascular function. A small incision in the skin is made, and the time it takes for bleeding to stop (i.e., the bleeding time) is noted and recorded.

- Normal values: 1 to 9 minutes for the most common test type (Ivy)
- Conditions affecting test results: Decreased platelet count, uremia, high blood levels of aspirin or indomethacin, high doses of warfarin (Coumadin).
- Special nursing considerations:
    1. Do not use the arm adjacent to a mastectomy.
    2. Assess if the client is taking salicylates, warfarin, or indomethacin.
    3. Following the test, apply pressure to incision site.

Test: Blood urea nitrogen (BUN)

Urea is a metabolite of protein metabolism. It is produced in the liver, where free ammonia is formed. It is transported in the blood to the kidneys, where it is excreted. Because both the liver and kidneys are involved, the BUN is an excellent measure of their function.

- Normal values: 10 to 20 mg/dl in adults
- Conditions affecting test results: Late pregnancy, heavy intake of protein, overhydration and dehydration, and drugs such as aminoglycosides, nephrotoxic agents, and some antibiotics.

- Special nursing considerations:
    1. Tell the client that fasting is not required.
    2. Explain the procedure and the test results to the client.
    3. Collect a current medication history and forward to laboratory.

Test: Complete blood count (CBC)

A CBC measures a variety of blood components: red blood cells (RBCs), white blood cells (WBCs), hemoglobin, hematocrit, platelet count, and a differential count of RBCs and WBCs.

- Normal values:

    RBC--4.5 to 6 million/mm^3 in male adults
    4.2 to 5.4 million/mm^3 in female adults
    WBC--5,000 to 10,000/mm^3
    Hemoglobin--14 to 18 g/dl in male adults
    12 to 16 g/dl in female adults
    Hematocrit--42% to 52% in male adults
    37% to 47% in female adults
    Platelet count--150,000 to 400,000/mm^3 in adults

- Conditions affecting test results: Hemorrhage, pregnancy, living at high altitudes, hydration state, and some drugs.
- Special nursing considerations:
    1. Explain the procedure and reason for the test.
    2. Assess history of drugs being taken and where client lives.
    3. Assess health history.

Test: Coombs' test, indirect

This test detects antibodies against red blood cells. The test is done prior to blood transfusion and in a pregnant woman if she is Rh negative and her fetus is Rh positive.

A sample of the client's blood is mixed with a special solution containing antibodies to human antibodies. Agglutination of the RBCs indicates a positive result.

- Normal values: Negative--no agglutination
- Conditions affecting test results: Insulin, chlorpromazine (Thorazine), penicillins, phenytoin (Dilantin), tetracyclines, and levodopa.
- Special nursing considerations:
    1. Assess medications the client is taking.
    2. Explain the procedure and meaning of test results.
    3. Tell that client that fasting is not required.

Test: Creatinine

Creatinine is a metabolite excreted entirely by the kidneys, making its level an excellent measure of renal function. Elevations of creatinine occur only in kidney disease. This test, along with the blood urea nitrogen (BUN), make up the "renal function studies."

- Normal values:

    0.6 to 1.2 mg/dl in adult males

    0.5 to 1.1 mg/dl in adult females

    Any value greater than 4.0 indicates serious renal function impairment.

- Conditions affecting test results: Some drugs, such as chemotherapeutic agents and aminoglycosides, and nephrotoxic medications.
- Special nursing considerations:
    1. Assess medications the client is taking.
    2. Discuss test results with the client.

Test: Erythrocyte sedimentation rate

This nonspecific test detects infectious, inflammatory, and cancer processes. It is often prescribed for clients with vague symptoms and is used to monitor client response to intervention therapies. In many diseases, the plasma protein increases, causing red blood cells to pile up on one another, increasing their weight. This causes them to fall faster when blood is allowed to stand after being drawn. The speed of this descent is called the sed rate.

- Normal values: up to 15 mm/hour in adult males

    up to 20 mm/hour in adult females

- Conditions affecting test results: Pregnancy, menstruation, oral contraceptives, aspirin, cortisone, and vitamin A.
- Special nursing considerations:
    1. Assess medications the client is taking.
    2. Do not let collected blood stand longer than 3 hours before testing. Be sure blood sample is sent to the laboratory immediately after being drawn.

Test: Glucose (fasting blood sugar)

This test is used to diagnose diabetes mellitus and to monitor blood glucose levels in clients with diabetes.

- Normal values: 70 to 110 mg/dl in adults
- Conditions affecting test results: Trauma, infection, myocardial infarction, cerebrovascular accident, and some drugs.

- Special nursing considerations:
    1. Have the client fast for at least 12 hours.
    2. Assess health history for current complaints.
    3. Do not give insulin or oral hypoglycemics until blood is drawn.

Test: Glycosylated hemoglobin (HBA$_{1c}$)

This test is used to evaluate long-term blood glucose control. The A$_{1c}$ components of hemoglobin have glucose attached to them (glycosylated) that is not diluted in the bloodstream. The amount of glucose attached is dependent on the amount of circulating glucose. Therefore, since red blood cells live approximately 120 days, the average blood glucose level for that period can be determined.
- Normal values: 4% to 8%
- Conditions affecting test results: Sickle cell anemia, chronic kidney disease, and late pregnancy.
- Special nursing considerations
    1. No special nursing considerations.

Test: Pregnancy

The human chorionic gonadotropic (hCG) hormone is secreted into the blood and urine after an ovum is fertilized. It can appear as early as 10 days after conception. There are four types of tests: biologic, immunologic, radioreceptor assay, and radioimmunoassay. Each type detects the presence of HCG, which indicates only that there is a pregnancy, not that it is a *normal* pregnancy.
- Normal values: Positive only if the client is pregnant
- Conditions affecting test results: Blood or protein in the urine can give false-positive results, as can diuretics, tranquilizers, hypnotics, and anticonvulsants.
- Special nursing considerations:
    1. Teach the client to collect a first-void in the morning as it has the greatest concentration of HCG.
    2. Tell the client that fasting is not required.
    3. Provide prenatal teaching if the test is positive.

Test: Prothrombin time (PT)

This test evaluates the clotting mechanism. When there is a decreased amount of clotting factor, the PT is prolonged. To assure uniform reporting results, the World Health Organization has established the international normalized ratio (INR) value. Many institutions report both the INR and absolute numbers.

- Normal values: 11.0 to 12.5 seconds; 85% to 100%: INR therapeutic level--2.0 to 3.5
- Conditions affecting test results: Alcohol, high-fat diet, vitamin K, heparin, salicylates, and some antibiotics.
- Special nursing considerations:
  1. Assess medications the client is taking.
  2. If the client is taking warfarin, hold morning dose until blood is drawn.

Electrocardiogram tests

Test: Ambulatory monitoring (Holter monitor)

A client undergoing this test wears electrocardiogram (ECG) leads connected to a monitor that continuously records the heart's electrical activity. The monitor is worn all the time, during awake hours and during sleep. The client records daily activities and any symptoms of cardiac distress during the test. Usually the test is performed for 24 to 48 hours. The purpose of the test is to identify suspected heart rhythm abnormalities.

- Normal values: Normal sinus rhythm.
- Conditions affecting test results: The client's inability to cooperate with keeping leads in place.
- Special nursing considerations:
  1. Teach the client about the procedure and monitor.
  2. Explain the need to keep a careful diary of daily activities.
  3. Teach the client not to bathe or use electric hygiene equipment (razors, toothbrushes).
  4. Instruct the client to call if he had any difficulties with the electrodes, monitor, or daily activities.

Test: Cardiac exercise stress test

This test measures cardiac function while a client is doing some type of physical activity (stress), such as walking on a treadmill or riding a stationary bicycle. The speed and elevation of the physical activity is gradually increased while heart rate, blood pressure, and ECG are monitored. Thallium, dobutamine, or adenosine may be given if a client has limitations and cannot perform adequately to stress the heart.

- Normal values: Ability to maintain a cardiac rate that is 85% of maximum rate for age and gender without cardiac symptoms or ECG changes.

- Conditions affecting test results: Having a heavy food intake before test, nicotine ingestion, and drugs such as propranolol (Inderal) and digoxin.
- Special nursing considerations:
    1. Teach the client to not eat, drink, or smoke for 4 or 5 hours before test.
    2. Explain test risks to the client and get a signed informed consent.
    3. Explain that the client should wear loose clothing and good walking shoes for the test.
    4. Take pre-test vital signs to establish a baseline.

Fluid analysis

Test: Amniocentesis

Studying amniotic fluid provides vital information about a developing fetus. Genetic anomalies, fetal lung maturity, and fetal status are all evaluated using amniocentesis. The test requires puncturing the abdominal wall into the uterine cavity and withdrawing amniotic fluid.

- Normal values: Vary, depending on the reason for doing the test.
- Conditions affecting test results: None.
- Special nursing considerations:
    1. Provide emotional support to the mother and family, letting them express their fears and concerns.
    2. Assess the mother's vital signs and the fetal heart rate.
    3. Explain that she will feel a slight discomfort when the needle touches the uterus.
    4. Have the client lie on her left side if she experiences dizziness or nausea during the procedure.
    5. Tell the client to contact caregivers if she has any post-procedure pain, fever, or fetal hyperactivity.

Test: Thoracentesis

This test is performed when there is an accumulation of fluid in the pleural space (pleural effusion). It involves inserting a needle attached to a syringe into the pleural space to remove the fluid for analysis and to relieve dyspnea and pain associated with pleural pressure.

The removed fluid is analyzed for color and density, white blood cells, protein, glucose, and various enzymes. Studies may also be done to detect tumor cells in clients with known carcinoma.

- Normal values: Normal pleural fluid
- Conditions affecting test results: There are no conditions that have an adverse effect on this test.
- Special nursing considerations:
    1. Explain the procedure and reasons for doing it to the client.
    2. Have the client sign an informed consent as this is an invasive procedure.
    3. Teach the client not to move or cough during procedure. If coughing is a problem, give her a cough suppressant.
    4. Monitor vital signs and the client for complaints of discomfort, excessive sweating, and fainting during procedure.
    5. Post-procedure, monitor client for signs of pneumothorax (tachypnea, dyspnea, restlessness, decreased breath sounds).

Endoscopy

Test: Colonoscopy

The use of a fiberoptic colonoscope permits the entire colon, from anus to ileocecal valve, to be visualized. Polyps, inflammation, neoplasms, ulcers, and hemorrhage can be detected. The test is performed on any client who has positive occult blood stools, bowel habit changes, or lower gastrointestinal (GI) bleeding. Clients who have a family history of colon disease should be tested regularly.

- Normal values: Normal colon
- Conditions affecting test results: Poor bowel preparation and hemorrhage, both of which cloud the endoscope lens and restrict visualization.
- Special nursing considerations:
    1. Teach the client the importance of proper bowel preparation.
    2. Explain the procedure and reassure the client that privacy will be maintained.
    3. Teach the client that flatulence will be present and there may be some gas pains after the procedure.
    4. Encourage eating and forced fluids when client has recovered from the sedation and there is no evidence of bowel perforation.

Nuclear scans

Test: Bone scan

A radioactive isotope is injected into a peripheral vein and a scanning camera examines the skeletal system. This test is done to detect bone malignancies but also can help evaluate trauma or unexplained pain. If

pathology exists, there is an increased uptake of the radioactive isotope in the area of pathology.
- Normal values: No anomalies found
- Conditions affecting test results: Clients who are pregnant or lactating should not have this test because of risk to the fetus or infant.
- Special nursing considerations:
    1. Assure the client that there is no danger from the radioactive material.
    2. Explain that the procedure takes up to 3 hours to complete.
    3. Encourage the client to force fluids after the test to help excrete the isotope.

Test: Thyroid scan

This test evaluates the size and function of the thyroid gland. A radioactive isotope is taken by mouth and a nuclear scanner is passed over the thyroid gland. Any areas of increased or decreased uptake of the isotope indicate pathology. The test is an excellent diagnostic tool for detecting thyroid nodules.
- Normal values: No areas of increased or decreased uptake of the radioactive isotope. Gland is normal size and shape.
- Conditions affecting test results: Recent intake of iodine-containing foods, cough medicines, oral contraceptives, or multiple vitamins.
- Special nursing considerations:
    1. Assess the client for allergies to iodine.
    2. Explain the procedure and reassure the client that there will be no discomfort.
    3. Teach the client to restrict use of iodine-containing drugs and thyroid drugs.

Sputum test

Test: Sputum culture and sensitivity

Sputum culture helps identify pathogens in a client with respiratory infections. The sensitivity test is useful in determining the most appropriate antibacterial drug therapy.

To culture the specimen, sputum samples are smeared onto a culture medium and the resulting bacterial growth is analyzed, usually in 24 hours. To determine the sensitivity, the specimen is cultured in various liquid dilutions of drugs or on solid media containing various concentrations of drugs to determine susceptibility of client's bacterial infection to antibiotics or antibacterials.

- Normal values: Negative for pathogenic bacterial growth.
- Conditions affecting test results: Collection of saliva instead of sputum.
- Special nursing considerations:
    1. Give the client a sterile sputum container the night before the test.
    2. Teach the client how to cough up sputum from the lungs and not to put saliva in the container.
    3. Teach the client to rinse mouth with water before coughing up specimen.
    4. Tell the client to collect specimen the first thing in the morning before eating or drinking.
    5. Tell the client to collect at least a teaspoon of sputum.

Urine tests

Test: Urinalysis

Total urinalysis is a series of tests performed on a urine specimen. The specimen does not have to be a "clean-catch specimen," but if signs of urinary infection are evident, a mid-stream, clean-catch specimen may be advisable. Urinalysis studies color, clarity, odor, pH, specific gravity, protein, presence of crystals and blood cells, and ketones.

- Normal values:
    Appearance--clear
    Color--yellow
    Odor--sharp
    pH--average 6.0
    Specific gravity--1.005 to 1.030
    Protein--up to 8 mg/dl
    WBCs--0 to 4
    RBCs--no more than 2
    Negative for ketone, glucose, casts, crystals, and nitrites
- Conditions affecting test results: Foods such as carrots, beets, and asparagus, acidic or alkaline diet, and various drugs.
- Special nursing considerations:
    1. Assess the client's medication and dietary history.
    2. Teach the client how to do a mid-stream collection.
    3. Be sure specimen goes to the laboratory promptly.

X-ray exams

Test: Computed tomography (CT)

A CT scan is a non-invasive x-ray examination used to detect tumors, cysts, inflammation, perforations, ulcers, obstructions, and aneurysms. The CT image develops from passing x-rays through the body at various angles. Organ tissue density permits penetration at different densities, creating an image on a computer monitor. Various dyes enhance the image, which can be reproduced on Polaroid film.

- Normal values: No abnormalities
- Conditions affecting test results: Metallic objects that have not been removed, obesity over 300 pounds, bowel filled with fecal matter.
- Special nursing considerations:
    1. Assess the client's allergy history, especially to iodine.
    2. Explain the procedure to the client, emphasizing that his cooperation is essential to a successful test.
    3. Show the client the CT machine to help alleviate fear and any concern for claustrophobia.
    4. Keep the client NPO for 4 hours before test.
    5. Force fluids post-test, if dye had been used, to help eliminate it from the body.

Test: Magnetic resonance imaging (MRI)

In this non-invasive examination of various body organs and structures, the client is placed in a magnetic field and radio waves are passed through the body part. The test is beneficial in viewing bone and blood vessels that do not image well in CT. MRI has the advantage of not exposing the client to radiation. A disadvantage of MRI is the preclusion of clients who have metal implants, clips, pacemakers, or had major abdominal surgery within 6 weeks.

- Normal values: No abnormalities
- Conditions affecting test results: Movement during the scan.
- Special nursing considerations:
    1. Explain the procedure and show the client the scanner, if possible, to allay fears.
    2. Teach the client to not wear any metal jewelry, dental prostheses, watches, and other metal devices.
    3. Warn the client that a thumping sound will be heard during the procedure.

Skin test

Test: Tuberculin test

This test determines if a client has been infected with the tubercle bacillus, but it does not diagnose active tuberculosis (TB). A purified protein derivative (PPD) of the tuberculosis bacillus is injected under the skin. If there is an area of induration greater than 5 mm and redness at the injection site within 72 hours, the test is positive. If the induration is less than 5 mm, the test is negative, meaning the client has not been infected with the tubercle bacillus.

- Normal values: Negative
- Conditions affecting test results: None
- Special nursing considerations:
    1. Teach the client that the test will not cause TB.
    2. After injecting the PPD, circle the resulting skin wheal with a marker.
    3. Read results in 72 hours, measuring the area of induration, not redness.
    4. Notify the client's health care provider if the test is positive.

HEALTH SCREENING

Health screening is a wellness philosophy of testing individuals to detect early symptoms of, or risk factors for, certain diseases, so that intervention may be instituted as soon as possible. Guidelines for the use of these screening tests are issued by various organizations, and change as new information is available. This section discusses the common and widely accepted recommendations for health screening tests. Individual practitioners may modify these recommendations based on a variety of factors specific to a client, i.e., presence of a positive family history or other predisposing risk factors.

Cancer

SUMMARY OF AMERICAN CANCER SOCIETY RECOMMENDATIONS FOR THE EARLY DETECTION OF CANCER IN ASYMPTOMATIC PEOPLE[1]			
Test	**Sex**	**Age**	**Frequency**
Sigmoidoscopy, preferably flexible	M & F	50 and over	Every 3 to 5 years
Fecal occult blood test	M & F	50 and over	Every year
Digital rectal exam	M & F	40 and over	Every year
Prostate-specific antigen (PSA)	M	50 and over	Every year
Papanicolaou (Pap) smear	F	All women who are, or who have been, sexually active or have reached age 18, should have an annual Pap test and pelvic examination. After a woman has had three or more consecutive satisfactory normal annual examinations, this test may be done less often at her caregiver's discretion.	
Breast self-examination	F	20 and over	Every month
Breast clinical examination	F	20 to 40 Over 40	Every 3 years Every year
Mammography	F	40 to 49 50 and over	Every 1 to 2 years Every year

[1]Modified from www.cancer.org/frames.html

Sigmoidoscopy
Description
Screening sigmoidoscopy is the passing of a lighted instrument
through the anal orifice into the sigmoid colon to detect pathology
(e.g. polyps, tumors, ulcerations). It also permits biopsy of suspicious
lesions. A flexible fiberoptic sigmoidoscope permits examination
about twice as far (16 to 20 inches) beyond the anus, as does the rigid
sigmoidoscope, but generally is more comfortable.

Rationale
Use of lighted scopes allows direct visualization of the lower bowel.
When performed on a recommended schedule, sigmoidoscopy permits
early detection of abnormalities, allowing for intervention at an early
stage in a disease process, i.e., removal of pre-cancerous polyps,
offering the client a better prognosis.

Normal values
The mucosa of the anal canal, rectum, and sigmoid colon should
appear normal.

Key nursing considerations and rationales
1. Explain the purpose of the test and the procedure.
   *Knowledge of how the test is conducted will help to alleviate
   anxiety.*
2. Teach the client how to do a proper bowel preparation, as
   ordered.
   *Screening sigmoidoscopies are most often done on an outpatient
   basis, and the client (or family) needs to know exactly how to do
   the bowel prep. The mucosa of the colon must be free of fecal
   matter to allow good visualization. Types of preps differ between
   clinicians, but generally include warm tap water or Fleet's enemas
   on the morning of the test until colon is clear. Some clinicians may
   require intestinal lavage, using polyethylene glycol electrolyte
   solution (GoLYTELY) and a pre-procedure liquid diet that is
   usually reserved for colonoscopies.*
3. Evaluate the client's ability to assume the knee-chest position.
   *If the client is having a rigid sigmoidoscopy, this is the required
   position. If the client is physically unable to assume this position,
   the physician must be notified.*
4. Explain to the client that gas pains, cramping, and the urge to
   defecate are normal sensations.
   Air may be introduced into the colon during the procedure; the

sigmoidoscope distends the colon, stimulating the defecation reflex.

5. Have the client practice slow, deep breathing and relaxation of the abdominal muscles.
   These techniques can reduce the discomfort he may experience during the procedure.

6. Help the client do breathing and relaxation during the exam.
   Anxiety may prevent client from performing these techniques without encouragement.

7. Monitor vital signs after the procedure.
   A vaso-vagal reaction may occur (decreased blood pressure, bradycardia, pallor, diaphoresis, nausea, syncope, and possible loss of consciousness).

8. Explain that passing a lot of flatus after the procedure is to be expected.
   Air introduced into the bowel during the procedure must be expelled.

9. Caution the client that passing small amounts of blood in the stool is normal, but to report any large amount of blood to the health care provider immediately.
   A biopsy, polypectomy, or trauma to the mucosa from the sigmoidoscope can cause small amounts of bleeding. Larger quantities of blood may be a symptom of bowel perforation (other symptoms include pain, abdominal distention, fever, and a general feeling of weakness).

Fecal occult blood test
Description

This test detects the iron-containing portion of the hemoglobin molecule (heme) in the stool. In most cases, the client can do it at home using a commercial test packet.

Normally, only very small amounts of blood are passed through the GI tract. Tumors and ulcerations can produce minute amounts of blood that is not overtly detectable in the stool. The use of special testing slides or tablets can easily detect any occult or hidden blood in the stool.

Small samples of fecal material from the center of two different areas of the stool are smeared on special guaiac-containing paper, per directions on the package. For the most accurate results, this should be repeated 3 days in a row. The client then mails the three samples in an envelope provided to the health care provider or a laboratory, where the samples are tested for the presence of occult blood.

Rationale
Small amounts of blood from intestinal lesions may be mixed with fecal material. The blood undergoes alteration during passage through the intestines and may not be recognizable as blood to the naked eye. Annual testing for fecal occult blood increases the likelihood of detecting a lesion in its earliest stages.

Normal values
There should be no occult blood in any of the stool specimens. Even one positive result requires further evaluation.

Key nursing considerations and rationales
1. Evaluate the client's understanding of, and ability to adhere precisely to, the manufacturer's instructions for collecting and mailing the specimens.
   Deviation from the accepted procedure decreases the reliability of the results.
2. Evaluate the client's diet and medications to eliminate (for 48 hours prior to, and during, the test) those that cause false-positive results.
   Foods causing false-positive results include rare meat, poultry, salmon, sardines, turnips, melons, and horseradish. Medications causing false-positive results include salicylates, iron, vitamin C, steroids, indomethacin (Indocin), and warfarin (Coumadin).
3. Advise the client not to take the stool specimens when there is bleeding from hemorrhoids or menstruation.
   Blood from hemorrhoids or menstruation may contaminate the stool, causing false-positive results.

Digital rectal exam
Description
In a digital rectal exam, the examiner inserts his gloved finger into the rectum to feel the rectal mucosa, get a stool sample, and (in men) palpate the prostate gland.

Rationale
For both men and women, digital rectal exam is another screening test

for colon cancer, as it lets the examiner feel for anything unusual in the lining of the rectum and remove a small amount of fecal material for testing for occult blood. In the male, it also permits palpation of the prostate gland for nodules and masses, which may be an indication of prostate cancer.

Normal values

The rectal wall should be free of palpable masses. The fecal material should be negative for occult blood. The prostate gland should feel round, with a groove between the two lobes. It should be firm, with no palpable nodules or masses.

Key nursing considerations and rationales

1. Explain the procedure to the client.
   Some clients find the procedure embarrassing, and a matter-of-fact explanation may help alleviate embarrassment and anxiety.

Prostate-specific antigen (PSA)

Description

The PSA test is performed on a venous blood sample, usually about 10 ml. It is used both to screen for prostate cancer (the level increases as the tumor load increases) and to evaluate response to treatment (the level decreases if surgery, chemotherapy, and/or radiation therapy are successful).

Rationale

PSA is a protein substance normally produced by the prostate gland. The level increases in the presence of prostate cancer, allowing evaluation of the severity of the cancer.

Normal values

0 to 4 ng/ml

Key nursing considerations and rationales

1. Explain purpose and procedure for the test; give the client time to discuss his anxiety.
   Most clients will be anxious not about the blood draw itself (although that is possible) but about the implications of the results. Talking with him about his fears may reduce them.
2. Explain that elevations in PSA may occur with prostatic conditions other than cancer.

Conditions that may elevate the PSA levels include benign prostatic hyperplasia, prostatitis, prostate surgery, and massage of the prostate (as during digital rectal exam).

Papanicolaou (Pap) smear
Description
A Pap smear is obtained during pelvic examination. A vaginal speculum is inserted and cells are removed from the cervical os by scraping with a small wooden spatula. A cervical brush is then rotated in the cervical os to remove cells. For women who have had a hysterectomy, the cells are obtained from the vaginal cuff. The cells are smeared on a glass slide and sprayed with or immersed in a fixative. Cytological (cell) examination is completed in a laboratory.

Rationale
Pap smears, when obtained and read accurately, have been found to reliably identify cellular changes indicative of pre-cancers and cancers. When performed on a regular basis, Pap smears can identify cellular changes in the early stages, facilitating early treatment. The prognosis is excellent when cellular changes are discovered and treated early.

Normal values
There should be no abnormal or atypical cells identified.

Key nursing considerations and rationales
1. Explain the purpose and procedure for the test.
   Pelvic examination itself can be an embarrassing and anxiety-producing procedure for some women. Concern about the results of the Pap smear will add to that anxiety. Specific information about the test will alleviate some anxiety.
2. Tell the client to not douche for 72 hours prior to the exam.
   Douching flushes away cellular material.
3. Assess the client for use of vaginal suppositories or jellies, presence of infection, and current menses.
   All of these factors can interfere with test results.
4. Have the client empty her bladder and bowel prior to the exam.
   Pressure on a full bladder or bowel during the exam will cause discomfort and, possibly, inadvertent evacuation. An empty bladder and bowel make the exam easier for the practitioner.
5. Provide privacy for the client; drape her appropriately.

Attending to the client's privacy and modesty needs helps to increase her comfort level.
6. Help the client relax during the examination.
   Muscle relaxation reduces the discomfort the speculum may cause.
7. Provide emotional support to the client who gets a report of an abnormal test.
   Clients getting a diagnosis of cancer or a precancerous condition become very frightened and need emotional support.

Breast self-examination (BSE)
Description
BSE is the client's systematic self-assessment of her breasts. It involves inspection and palpation.

Rationale
Within the health care community, there is controversy as to the efficacy of BSE in decreasing the mortality associated with breast cancer. Those who advocate BSE (among them the American Cancer Society) believe that with regular examination of the breasts, women will find most lesions at a stage where treatment would be most likely to effect a cure, thus decreasing mortality. BSE is recommended as an important screening tool.

Normal values
"Normal" breast tissue differs widely from person to person. In general, however, once a woman has become familiar with the appearance and texture of her own breasts, normal is considered to be no change from the usual.

Key nursing considerations and rationales
1. Teach the client the correct techniques of BSE. Have her perform in your presence.
   Correct technique is necessary to maximize the accuracy of the examination; having the client demonstrate the procedure is the best way to ensure that learning has occurred.
2. Explain to a premenopausal client that she should examine her breasts 5 to 10 days after the start of her menses.
   During this portion of the menstrual cycle the effects of hormones on the breast tissue are diminished.
3. Encourage the postmenopausal client to select 1 day each month on which to perform BSE.

This establishes a way to remember to perform BSE when the client no longer has a menstrual cycle.

Breast clinical examination
Definition
Breast clinical examination (BCE) is the use of inspection and palpation by a health care professional to examine a client's breasts.

Rationale
Detecting breast abnormalities as early as possible in their development increases the likelihood that the treatment will be the least invasive possible with the best prognosis. Regular examination (see recommended schedule in table above) by a health care practitioner skilled in the technique of BCE is one of the elements (along with BSE and regular mammography) of an early detection program. Technique is essentially the same as in BSE.

Normal values
There is no one definition of "normal" with regard to BCE. The absence of abnormal findings such as dimpling, nipple inversion, an "orange peel" appearance to the skin, and suspicious masses constitutes a negative BCE. Suspicious masses are those that are unilateral, not tender, irregular in shape, fixed, and firm. Most masses found in breast tissue are not malignant, although further testing may be necessary to determine this with certainty.

Key nursing considerations and rationale
1. Explain the procedure to the client.
   Knowledge of what will be done helps decrease anxiety.
2. Drape the client for the minimal amount of exposure necessary.
   This preserves the client's privacy.
3. Reassure the client that the majority of breast masses are benign.
   This helps to decrease her anxiety.

Mammography
Description
Mammography is a special x-ray procedure that can detect breast masses before they are palpable during BSE or BCE. It involves compressing the breast between two clear plastic plates, once from the top and bottom of the breast, and once from side to side, with an

x-ray image taken in each position. The images are compared to previous mammograms when these are available.

Rationale

Because mammograms can detect breast masses that are too small (less than 1 cm) to be felt during BSE or BCE, they are important in the effort to detect cancers at a stage when treatment can be the least invasive and the most likely to produce a cure.

Normal values

A negative mammogram is one in which there is no evidence of a suspicious mass or of a change from previous mammograms. False negative results are possible, since mammograms do not detect lesions with 100% accuracy.

Key nursing considerations and rationales

1. Encourage the client to have mammograms on a regular basis.
   Regular mammograms, BSE, and BCE currently are the best methods of early breast cancer detection.
2. Advise the client to avoid the use of deodorant, powder, and perfume on the day of the mammogram.
   These interfere with the quality of the x-ray films.
3. Explain that compression of the breasts during the exam may be uncomfortable but is necessary to achieve the best possible quality in the films and lasts for only a few moments.
   Understanding the reason for, and duration of, the discomfort will help the client tolerate it.

Heart disease

Cholesterol and triglycerides

Description

Testing for cholesterol and triglyceride levels is performed on a blood sample. Usually the sample is obtained by venipuncture, but for cholesterol screening in community settings or home testing kits, a finger-stick sample is used. Testing for total cholesterol, high-density lipoproteins (HDL), low-density lipoproteins (LDL), and triglycerides is referred to as a lipid profile. While the total cholesterol measurement does not require fasting, measurement of the lipid profile does. A low-fat, high-fiber diet and exercise can often control cholesterol levels. If these measures fail, medications may be prescribed for high-risk clients. The medications must be used in conjunction with--never in place of--dietary modifications.

Cholesterol is the main fat contributing to arteriosclerotic circulatory disease. While cholesterol is necessary for the body to manufacture steroids and bile, excess levels bind to arterial walls, causing plaque and subsequent occlusion of the vessel. This test evaluates the level of circulating cholesterol in the blood. Its value can change significantly during the day, affected by posture or illness. Conditions affecting test results: liver disease or some drugs, including oral contraceptives, sulfonamides, and some antibiotics. Pregnancy will elevate cholesterol levels.

Rationale

Increased cholesterol and triglyceride levels are known to be risk factors for atherosclerosis and coronary heart disease. Low HDL levels and elevated LDL levels--even if the total cholesterol is within normal limits--are known to also be risk factors for coronary heart disease.

Normal values
1. Cholesterol: 140 to 199 mg/dl
2. HDL: > 50 mg/dl
3. LDL: < 130 mg/dl
4. Triglycerides: 35 to 160 mg/dl

Key nursing considerations and rationales
1. When testing includes measurement of triglycerides, advise the client to fast for at least 12 hours and to avoid alcohol for at least 24 hours prior to the test.
   Ingested fats and alcohol may increase triglyceride levels.
2. If testing is done in a local screening setting or by a home testing kit, refer the client with abnormal results for follow-up medical care.
   Clients with abnormal lipid profiles need to be followed on a regular basis by a health care professional.
3. Encourage clients with high cholesterol and/or triglyceride levels to adhere to dietary and exercise regimens.
   Exercise and a low-fat, high-fiber diet are often successful in decreasing blood lipid levels.
4. Advise clients on antilipemic medications that they are to be used

in conjunction with, not in place of, a low-fat, high-fiber diet. *Clients sometimes believe that taking the medication lets them eat whatever they like.*

Hypertension
Description
Hypertension is generally defined as blood pressure levels consistently greater than 140 mm Hg systolic and greater than 90 mm Hg diastolic. According to the American Heart Association (AHA), "Diagnosis of high blood pressure is based on the average of two or more readings taken at each of two or more visits after an initial screening."

Rationale
Hypertension is known to be a risk factor for heart failure, stroke, and kidney failure. Early detection and intervention can prevent or at least lessen the morbidity and mortality associated with this condition.

Normal values

CLASSIFICATION OF BLOOD PRESSURE OF ADULTS AGE 18 YEARS AND OLDER			
Category	Systolic (mm Hg)		Diastolic (mm Hg)
Optimal	<120	&	<80
Normal	<130	&	<85
High normal	130 to 139	&	85 to 89
Hypertension STAGE 1 (Mild)	140 to 159	or	90 to 99
STAGE 2 (Moderate)	160 to 179	or	100 to 109
STAGE 3 (Severe)	≥180	or	≥110

*From the Sixth Report, Joint National Committee on Detection, Evaluation, and Treatment of High Blood Pressure, 1997

Key nursing considerations and rationale

1. Explain to the client that two or more readings may be taken during each of two or more visits to the health care provider.
   A variety of factors can elevate blood pressure for a short time; two readings, taken at different times during the same visit and averaged, and taken at two or more visits, allows for more accurate diagnosis.
2. Encourage the client taking antihypertensive medications not to discontinue the medication without talking to the health care provider.
   Clients may think that they do not need the medication because they feel well.

Vision

Glaucoma

Description

Glaucoma is a group of ophthalmologic disorders characterized by increased intraocular pressure, leading to damage to the optic nerve, loss of visual field, and eventual blindness. Screening for glaucoma includes medical and ocular histories, ophthalmoscope examination, measurement of intraocular pressure by tonometry, and measurement of peripheral vision. Recommendations for testing differ, but in general, adults over 40 (over 35 for blacks) should be screened every 3 to 5 years. Clients with diabetes, a family history of glaucoma, or other risk factor, should be screened every 1 or 2 years, beginning at an earlier age.

Rationale

Glaucoma is asymptomatic until significant and irreversible, once damage has been done; yet, if found early and treated appropriately, blindness is almost always preventable. Glaucoma has no cure, but medication and/or surgery can control the condition.

Normal values

10 to 22 mm Hg

Key nursing considerations and rationales

1. Assure the client that the examination procedure is not painful.
   The cornea is anesthetized with eyedrops if the tonometer is to be placed against the eye.

2. Explain that glaucoma has no symptoms until significant damage
   has been done.
   Clients may not seek eye examinations if they have no symptoms.

Refractive errors, amblyopia, and strabismus
Description
The American Academy of Ophthalmology recommends an initial eye
exam by age 4, with subsequent exams every 2 years. Screening for
refractive errors (farsightedness and nearsightedness), amblyopia (lazy
eye), and strabismus (misalignment of the eyes caused by imbalance
of the extraocular muscles), can be done either by a primary health
care provider or through vision testing programs in schools, churches,
and various community programs.

Rationale
Refractive errors can cause eye strain or decreased vision. Untreated
amblyopia can lead to loss of vision. Strabismus is fairly common in
children and needs to be corrected to avoid double or blurred vision.
Screening is relatively easy and inexpensive.

Normal values
Normal visual acuity is 20/20. Symmetrical, coordinated movement of
the eyes, in the same direction, is normal.

Key nursing considerations and rationale
1. Explain to parents that vision screening helps detect anomalies that
   may cause future problems, including loss of vision.
   Understanding the reason for screening will increase compliance.
2. Explain to the parents and the child being tested that there is no
   pain or discomfort.
   *Knowing that the tests do not hurt decreases anxiety and increases
   cooperation.*

Scoliosis

Description
Scoliosis is a lateral curvature of the spine, usually manifesting itself
during preadolescence. The American Academy of Orthopaedic
Surgeons and the Scoliosis Research Society recommend screening for
scoliosis in schools, although this recommendation is not universally
accepted. Currently these groups recommend screening girls in grades
5 and 7, and boys in grade 8 or 9. Screening is accomplished through

informed observation, i.e., the observer must know what to look for. The exam consists of viewing a child wearing only underpants from the rear, looking for symmetry of shoulders, scapulae, flanks, and hips. The child then bends forward, with the trunk parallel to the floor and the arms hanging free, as the examiner again assesses for symmetry.

Rationale

Those who advocate screening believe that finding scoliosis early in its development increases the likelihood that bracing, rather than surgery, will correct the curvature. The grade recommendations are based on the facts that girls reach adolescence earlier than boys and require treatment for scoliosis much more frequently than boys.

Normal values

Shoulder, scapulae, flank, and hip heights should be symmetrical.

Key nursing considerations and rationale

1. Provide for privacy for each child when performing screening. *Early adolescents are very private about their bodies and will be embarrassed to be examined in only their underpants.*

IMMUNIZATIONS

Overview

Immunization is the process of introducing antigens into the body to protect against infectious diseases. It may be *active,* giving a vaccine or toxoid to stimulate the immune system, or *passive,* giving immune globulins or antitoxins from immune persons or animals to nonimmune persons.

Some vaccines are administered prior to probable exposure, as to a person traveling to areas where cholera or typhoid are prevalent. Others are recommended for specific people at certain times of the year, i.e., the influenza and pneumococcal vaccines. Still other are recommended for all children, beginning shortly after birth. These immunization recommendations change as new information and new vaccines become available. Nurses are often responsible for the administration of vaccines and need to be knowledgeable about them.

Key nursing considerations and rationale

1. Encourage parents to complete the immunizations according to recommended schedules.
   Although these immunizations may be given later than recommended, children are at greatest risk for contracting infectious diseases during the first 2 years of life.

2. Explain to parents the risks of both the disease and the vaccine.
   Some people have fears about alleged adverse effects of vaccines, but these fears are not supported by scientific evidence. Even where adverse effects may be serious, the morbidity and mortality associated with contracting the disease usually is greater.

3. Assess parents' understanding of the written materials available for each vaccine from the U.S. Public Health Service.
   These pamphlets are written at a reading level that may not be understood by many parents.

4. Teach about the community resources that offer the vaccines at no or low cost.
   Many parents are not able to afford the health care provider visits necessary to complete all immunizations.

5. Teach parents how to keep a record of immunizations for each child, including the name and address of the person administering the vaccine.
   This provides information needed if the child is ever cared for by a different health care provider.

6. Assess for a history of any allergic reaction to a previous vaccine.
   Some reactions, i.e., anaphylaxis or severe illness, contraindicate subsequent doses of that vaccine.

7. Inform parents that acetaminophen (Tylenol) may be given for fever or pain.
   These are reactions that are not unusual following administration of some vaccines. Some practitioners recommend that acetaminophen be given just prior to administration of the diphtheria, tetanus, pertussis (DTP) vaccine, followed by two more doses at 4- to 6-hour intervals, since this vaccine commonly produces inflammation at the injection site and a low-grade fever.

8. Assess for HIV infection or any other immune-deficient state in the child or a close household member before administering oral poliovirus (OPV).
   Persons with decreased immune competence are at risk for developing vaccine-associated paralysis because live virus is used in the OPV.

9. Read package inserts for all vaccines to be administered. *Vaccines from different manufactures may need to be handled differently; even from the same manufacturer, information about vaccines may change over time.*

RECOMMENDED CHILDHOOD IMMUNIZATION SCHEDULE
UNITED STATES, 1998[1]

Vaccine	Birth	1 mo.	2 mos.	4 mos.	6 mos.	12 mos.	15 mos.	18 mos.	4-6 yrs.	11-12 yrs.	14-16 yrs.
Hepatitis B (HBV)	HBV #1										
		HBV #2			HBV #3						
Diphtheria, tetanus, pertussis (DTaP or DTP)			√	√	√			√	√	Td (Tetanus and diphtheria)	
Haemophilus influenzae type b (Hib)			√	√	√	√					
Polio			√	√		√			√		
Measles, mumps, rubella (MMR)							√		√		
Varicella							√				

[1]Adapted from www.aap.org/family/parents/immunize.htm

CHAPTER 3

Restoring Wellness

SHOCK

Overview

Shock is a reduction in circulating blood volume causing an inadequate delivery of oxygen and nutrients to the body's cells. Cell death can occur because of the reduced perfusion.

Shock is classified according to its cause. Since it can result from a variety of causes, nursing care is primarily directed toward ongoing assessment of clients at risk to recognize the symptoms early and begin interventions as soon as possible. Once the shock state has developed, intensive nursing care is required.

Classifications of shock

1. Cardiogenic shock--occurs because of the heart's impaired ability to function as a pump. Consequently, the cardiac stroke volume is reduced and cardiac output decreased. Blood pressure falls, and tissue perfusion does not meet cellular demands. Clinical conditions that may cause cardiogenic shock include myocardial infarction, dysrhythmias, and heart failure.
2. Hypovolemic shock--occurs when the intravascular volume decreases relative to the size of the vascular system. Circulating blood volume decreases, as well as venous return to the heart. Cardiac stroke volume is lessened, cardiac output is decreased, blood pressure falls, and tissue perfusion does not meet cellular demands. Clinical conditions that may cause hypovolemic shock include hemorrhage, dehydration, burns, vomiting, diarrhea, diuresis, ascites, and surgery.
3. Distributive shock--occurs when massive vasodilation lets blood pool in peripheral blood vessels. Even though there is no actual loss of fluid from the vascular system, the pooling of blood in the periphery causes decreased blood return to the heart, causing decreased stroke volume, decreased cardiac output, and consequent decreased tissue perfusion.
   There are three types of distributive shock:
   a. Anaphylactic shock--the vasodilation is the result of histamine release caused by an allergic reaction to an insect bite, food, drugs, etc.
   b. Neurogenic shock--the vasodilation is the result of decreased sympathetic nervous system tone, caused by such things as spinal cord injury, spinal anesthesia, drugs that depress the nervous system, and insulin reaction.
   c. Septic shock--the vasodilation is the result of massive infection,

most often by gram-negative bacteria. Septic shock has two phases: hyperdynamic (warm shock) and, as the shock state progresses, hypodynamic (cold shock).

4. Obstructive shock--occurs from some physical obstruction to the blood flow, which causes decreased cardiac output and decreased tissue perfusion, even though the heart pumps normally and there is no reduction in intravascular volume. Causes of obstructive shock include cardiac tamponade, tension pneumothorax, pulmonary embolism, and dissecting aortic aneurysm.

Pathophysiology

1. All types of shock cause some disruption to blood flow, to the heart's pumping ability, and/or to vascular tone.
2. At first, those parts of the circulatory system not initially affected compensate to maintain tissue perfusion. Ultimately, the volume of blood reaching the tissues decreases, so fewer nutrients and less oxygen reach the cells. Lacking oxygen, the cells metabolize anaerobically, causing an accumulation of lactic acid and metabolic acidosis.
3. The accumulating carbon dioxide produces increased levels of carbonic acid, leading to hyperventilation and subsequent respiratory alkalosis. Cellular permeability increases, and cellular structures are damaged, resulting in cellular death and multiple organ failure.

Key assessments and rationales

Note: For the most part, nursing assessments are applicable to all classes of shock. Specific mention will be made when assessments are specific to one class.

1. Get a complete history of any adverse reaction to medications, food, diagnostic imaging contrast media, iodine, fish (anaphylactic shock).
   A history of any previous allergic reaction must be communicated to all personnel who will be involved in the client's care.
2. Do a complete physical assessment of all clients at risk for developing shock.
   Provides a baseline against which to measure variations.
3. Perform ongoing physical assessments, paying close attention to changes in level of consciousness, skin and body temperature, urinary output, heart rate, respiratory rate and depth, blood pressure, and bowel sounds.
   Detecting shock at the compensatory stage greatly improves the client's prognosis. Assessing all body systems is necessary to

ascertain the effects of treatment, progression of the shock state, and deterioration in organ functioning.

4. Assess the client's and family's emotional state and coping mechanisms.
   Fear and anxiety are common responses to a life-threatening condition.

Key interventions and rationales

Note: Nursing intervention are, for the most part, applicable to all classifications of shock. Specific mention will be made when interventions are specific to one class.

1. Monitor hemodynamic status and report any changes promptly.
   Deviations from the client's baseline normal values are important indicators. Noting them early and instituting treatment immediately improve the client's chances of survival.

2. Maintain airway patency and administer oxygen as prescribed.
   Adequate exchange of oxygen and carbon dioxide in the pulmonary-capillary bed is necessary to maximize the delivery of oxygen to the cells and the removal of carbon dioxide.

3. Administer intravenous (I.V.) fluids. Monitor for complications
   Crystalloids (commonly Ringer's lactate and 0.9% sodium chloride) and colloids (e.g., albumin, dextran) are used to replace vascular volume in all types of shock. Blood products are administered in hypovolemic shock caused by hemorrhage. The nurse must monitor fluid replacement carefully for therapeutic response (including urinary output, vital signs, and skin perfusion) and for complications (including pulmonary edema and circulatory overload).

4. Turn and position the client frequently and cautiously.
   Decreased skin perfusion predisposes the client to skin breakdown. Sudden, rapid position changes in shock clients can cause fluid shift and worsen shock condition.

5. Maintain strict asepsis. Monitor for infection.
   Clients in shock have numerous invasive procedures performed, increasing the likelihood of infection. The nurse must be sure that the client's care follows infection control policies to decrease the chance of septic shock developing. If an infection does develop, identifying it in its earliest stages improves the prognosis.

6. Maintain normal body temperature.
   Excessive heat and cold with shivering increase the heart's workload.

7. Explain all procedures and changes in client status to the client and family in terms they can understand.
   Simple, clear, and timely explanations will help decrease the fear and anxiety the client and family experience. If the shock state becomes irreversible, the family needs support and understanding as they come to grips with the likelihood of death.

Drugs commonly used in this disorder
1. Dopamine hydrochloride (Intropin) is a vasopressor and inotropic agent that is used in shock to increase blood pressure, cardiac output, and urine output. Dose range: 0.5 to 2 mcg/kg/minute I.V. to increase renal blood flow; 2 to 10 mcg/kg/minute I.V. to both increase renal blood flow and stimulate the heart. Doses >10 mcg/kg/minute may decrease renal blood flow. Nursing considerations include monitoring hemodynamic measurements, urine output, and peripheral pulses during administration and titrating flow rate to maintain within preset parameters; using large vein for administration; using infusion pump; assessing I.V. site frequently for extravasation.
2. Nitroprusside (Nipride, Nitropress) is a vasodilator used to produce peripheral vasodilation, thereby decreasing preload and afterload in cardiogenic shock. Dose range: 0.3 to 10 mcg/kg/minute I.V. Nursing considerations include monitoring hemodynamic measurements, urine output, and peripheral pulses during administration and titrating flow rate to maintain within preset parameters; protecting fluid from light by wrapping infusion bottle in aluminum foil; using infusion pump.
3. Cimetidine (Tagamet) is a histamine H_2 antagonist that is used to both prevent and treat stress-induced upper GI ulcers and bleeding in shock states and other critical illnesses. Dose range: 50 mg/hour continuous I.V.; 300 mg I.V. q6h. Nursing considerations include assessing for GI pain or bleeding, fecal occult blood; assessing elderly or debilitated client for confusion.

Nutrition considerations
1. Caloric requirements increase to over 3,000 per day because of increased metabolic rate.
2. Enteral feedings via nasogastric or gastrostomy tube are preferred, if possible and tolerated.

VIEW THE TWO PROGRAMS *"ACID/BASE BALANCE"* AND *"FLUID ELECTROLYTE BALANCE"* BEFORE PROCEEDING. THESE ARE THE 2ND AND 3RD PROGRAMS ON THE VIDEO MODULE.

IMMOBILITY

Overview

Immobility is the temporary or permanent loss of motor function, sensory function, or a combination of the two. The loss of the ability to move body parts or experience sensation presents hazards to a client's well-being because immobility affects all body systems. Most sequelae of immobility can be prevented with good nursing care.

Causes of immobility

1. Trauma--most commonly severed nerve or muscle pathways and fractures.
2. Degenerative pathology--arthritis, myasthenia gravis, multiple sclerosis, and some poisonings.
3. Cellular anoxia--from hemorrhage, vascular occlusion, or acid/base imbalances.
4. Medical interventions--surgery, casting to immobilize joints.
5. Psychopathology--severe anxiety and some forms of psychosis.

Results of immobility

1. Loss of motor function--muscle weakness, paralysis, and muscle atrophy.
2. Loss of sensory function--full or partial blindness, deafness, anesthesias, paresthesias, and full or partial aphasia.
3. Equilibrium--positional, weight, and postural distortions and disturbances, such as not knowing what position a limb is in.

Nursing goals in immobility

1. Maintaining function in unaffected body parts.
2. Regaining optimum function in parts affected.
3. Restoring client to a functional role in society.

Nursing interventions

1. Teach and encourage deep-breathing exercises to prevent respiratory complications.
2. Change position frequently, maintaining correct body alignment, to prevent contractures and stasis ulcers.

3. Promote good general hygiene to prevent infection.
4. Increase fluid intake to 3,000 ml per day to prevent constipation and urinary tract infections (UTIs). Use juices and high-fiber foods.
5. Weigh the client regularly to detect any weight loss from inadequate nutrition.
6. Teach the client active range-of-motion exercises to maintain muscle strength. Perform passive range-of-motion to maintain joint mobility.
7. Regularly perform neurovascular and neurological checks to evaluate any circulatory complications and altered perceptions.
8. Provide emotional support to the client and family to reduce anxiety, fear, and depression.
9. Refer the client to support groups and vocational counseling to build self-esteem and develop new skills.

BLOOD TRANSFUSION

Overview

Blood replacement or transfusion is the administration of whole blood, packed red cells, plasma, platelets, or other components. Blood replacement is done to:
1. replace blood loss from trauma, hemorrhage, or surgery.
2. maintain hemoglobin and increase red cells in severe anemia.
3. replace lost blood components, i.e., platelets, clotting factors.

The source of blood being transfused may be autologous (the client's own blood) or homologous (a donor's blood). Autologous transfusions generally are safer because they decrease the chance of transfusion reactions. Homologous transfusions carry the risk of transfusion reactions and the client becoming infected with hepatitis viruses or HIV.

The procedure for transfusing blood is a nursing responsibility. Assessing and monitoring the client and regulating the transfusion process must be carefully controlled to assure safe administration and client protection.

Key assessments and rationales
1. Assess the client's understanding of the reason for the transfusion and whether a previous transfusion had been given.

If the client has had previous transfusions of blood products, there is less likelihood of a transfusion reaction. The client may be anxious about the procedure; assessing his knowledge level will help you determine how much reassurance he may need.

2. Establish baseline vital signs.
   Any change in the vital signs during the transfusion could indicate a reaction. Baselines are needed to measure changes.

3. Make sure that a signed consent form is in the client's record and that the client knows the signs of a transfusion reaction.
   A signed consent form is required because the procedure is an invasive one. The client should know the signs of a transfusion reaction so they can be reported early.

Key interventions and rationales

1. Check the identity of the client, the blood product, and the compatibility of the client and blood product with another RN.
   This assures the right client is getting the right product.

2. Assess the I.V. site for correct size needle, if I.V. is in place, what fluid is infusing, or if the site is suitable for the transfusion.
   The correct needle size for transfusions is 18 or 19 gauge. Anything smaller may cause clogging of the needle. An I.V. site should be selected that has a large vein and would be comfortable for the client. Blood should only run with NSS, preferably via a Y type transfusion set.

3. After transfusion is started, stay with the client for at least the first 15 or 30 minutes, monitoring vital signs every 10 or 15 minutes. Administer the first 50 ml slowly over at least 15 minutes.
   This is the period when most transfusion reactions occur. Limiting volume minimizes the severity of reaction if one occurs and allows reaction to be noted before larger amounts of blood are administered.

4. After the first 15 minutes, increase the transfusion rate to complete it within prescribed time (or as quickly as the client's condition permits).
   Blood must be infused within a maximum of 4 hours to maintain biologic effectiveness and limit risk of bacterial growth.

5. Observe the client every 15 minutes during the administration, taking vital signs as directed by hospital policy.
   Clients with cardiac conditions are in danger of fluid overload or, if the blood is administered rapidly, heart failure.

6. Document the administration, including the blood product given.
Provides continuity of care.

TRANSFUSION ADVERSE EFFECTS AND INTERVENTIONS		
Adverse reactions to blood administration can occur during the first 15 minutes of infusing and up to 2 hours after it has occurred.		
Reaction	**Signs and symptoms**	**Intervention**
Hemolytic	Fever, chills, nausea, flushing of face, tachycardia, dyspnea, pain, and severe anxiety	1. Stop transfusion. This is a life-threatening situation--keep I.V. line open with NSS. 2. Call health care provider. 3. Monitor for shock; take vital signs q15 minutes. 4. Monitor urine output for signs of decrease. 5. Return blood and delivery system to the laboratory along with samples of client's blood and urine.
Allergic	Headache, urticaria, chest pain, wheezing, hypotension, anxiety	Same as above. Request orders for and administer antihistamines as prescribed.
Circulatory overload	Dyspnea, cough, anxiety, crackles, tachycardia, orthopnea, increased venous pressure, distended neck veins, bounding pulse	1. Elevate head of bed to ease breathing. 2. Slow the transfusion. 3. Monitor vital signs q15 minutes. 4. Notify health care provider.
Sepsis	Chills, fever, low blood pressure, shock within 2 hours of transfusion	1. Stop transfusion--keep I.V. line open with NSS. 2. Monitor vital signs. 3. Take blood sample for culture. 4. Notify health care provider.

POSTOPERATIVE COMPLICATIONS

Overview
Complications may occur after any surgical procedure. They increase morbidity and mortality and increase the cost of health care. The nurse plays a vital role in preventing postoperative complications and in managing them if they occur.

Shock
Shock is one of the most serious postoperative complications. (See section on "Shock," page 50.)

Hemorrhage
Overview
Postoperative hemorrhage is classified as primary (at the time of surgery), intermediary (occurring during the first few hours after surgery as the return to normal blood pressure dislodges clots from untied vessels), and secondary (occurring later in the postoperative course as a result of insecure ligature tying, infection, or erosion of a blood vessel from a drainage tube).

Clinical manifestations
The physiological signs of hemorrhage depend on how much blood is lost how quickly. They usually appear in approximately the following order: apprehension and restlessness; thirst; pale, cool, moist skin; increased pulse; decreased temperature; rapid, deep respirations; decreased cardiac output; decreased blood pressure (arterial and venous); rapidly decreasing hemoglobin; pale lips and conjunctiva; ringing in the ears; progressive weakness; and death.

Key interventions and rationales
1. Administer sedatives or analgesics as ordered.
   Apprehension and restlessness increase metabolic rate, which increases bleeding.
2. Assess the incision for bleeding.
   The incision is the most evident site of bleeding, so it should be assessed first.
3. Administer blood/blood products as ordered.
   Blood and blood products are the best replacements for frank hemorrhage.

Deep vein thrombosis
Overview
Inflammation of a deep vein, with an accompanying blood clot, results from a number of factors that surround the surgical experience. These include too-tight leg holders, a blanket roll or prolonged "dangling," putting pressure on the popliteal space, loss of body fluids causing hemoconcentration, and decreased circulation because of decreased mobility and metabolism. The nurse has the primary role in preventing and treating deep vein thrombosis (DVT).

Clinical manifestations
Initially, the client may complain of pain or cramping in the calf, exacerbated by gentle compression. Within a day or two, there is painful swelling of the leg and the client may develop a low-grade fever, chills, and diaphoresis.

Key interventions and rationales
1. Preoperatively, teach the client and family leg exercises.
   Preop teaching will encourage compliance with postop exercises.
2. Assess for Homans' sign. Measure calf circumference and compare to unaffected leg.
   Pain on dorsiflexion of the foot with the knee bent is an early sign of DVT. Swelling can be picked up earlier than visualization.
3. Apply and monitor compression device(s) as prescribed.
   External compression applied from toes to groin using elastic bandages, antiembolic stockings, and/or pneumatic compression devices help prevent stasis of blood.
4. Administer and monitor anticoagulant therapy as ordered.
   Parenteral and/or oral anticoagulants are used both prophylactically and after a DVT has occurred.
5. Maintain adequate hydration and encourage early ambulation.
   This prevents venous stasis.

Pulmonary embolism
Overview
A pulmonary embolus (PE) occurs when a blood clot, air, amniotic fluid, or fat moves from its point of origin, through the bloodstream, to the pulmonary arterial system. After surgery, the primary sites for the development of a blood clot that can embolize are the pelvic and deep calf veins. The embolus causes some obstruction of the pulmonary arterial system, producing a ventilation-perfusion

mismatch, decreased oxygen and increased carbon dioxide levels, and sometimes pulmonary infarction. Complete obstruction causes profound respiratory and cardiovascular disturbances and may lead to sudden death.

Clinical manifestations

The size of the embolus and where it lodges in the pulmonary arterial system determine the severity of the symptoms. Sudden, often pleuritic, chest pain is usually present. Dyspnea, ranging from mild to very severe, is common. Other symptoms include tachypnea, tachycardia, anxiety, cough (perhaps with hemoptysis), wheezes, crackles, and pleural friction rub, and fever. If the embolism is large, shock symptoms may develop rapidly.

Key interventions and rationales

1. Encourage early ambulation, range-of-motion leg exercises, and use of leg compression devices after surgery.
   Prevention of DVT is the best prophylaxis for PE.
2. Administer oxygen.
   The ventilation/perfusion mismatch causes hypoxemia.
3. Administer pain medication as ordered.
   Chest pain increases anxiety, which leads to increased oxygen consumption.
4. Encourage deep breathing and coughing (suction if necessary).
   This assists in clearing respiratory secretions and preventing atelectasis.
5. Administer and monitor anticoagulant therapy as ordered.
   Initially, heparin will be administered by continuous I.V. to prevent the development of new thrombi. Warfarin (Coumadin) may follow if long-term therapy is needed.
6. Be prepared to administer and monitor thrombolytic drugs (streptokinase, urokinase).
   These drugs are used to dissolve emboli when the client is experiencing significant respiratory and cardiovascular consequences. Monitor the client carefully for bleeding.
7. Anticipate surgical intervention if PE is severe.
   Embolectomy (via thoracotomy or transvenous) may be indicated if the client is having significant symptoms or if there is a large obstruction of the pulmonary arterial system. Insertion of a Greenfield filter may be indicated if there are recurrent emboli.

Respiratory complications
Overview
Respiratory complications following surgery, especially abdominal and thoracic, are frequent and serious. They include atelectasis, hypoxemia, pneumonia, pleurisy, and superinfections. In elderly and debilitated clients, these complications are responsible for significant morbidity and mortality. The nurse's chief responsibility is preventing these complications.

Key interventions and rationales
1. Encourage frequent turning, deep breathing, coughing, and use of incentive spirometry (IS).
   These techniques promote lung expansion and mobilize secretions. If the client cannot mobilize secretions, suctioning may be needed.
2. Provide pain relief, preferably via patient-controlled analgesia (PCA).
   Pain decreases the client's ability to turn, deep breath, cough, and use IS. PCA promotes pain prevention, which is superior to pain relief, and gives the client a sense of control.
3. Promote early and consistent mobility.
   Mobility prevents stasis of secretions and improves lung expansion.
4. Perform frequent pulse oximetry.
   This provides information about oxygen saturation of the blood.

Urinary complications
Overview
Urinary complications following surgery may occur for many reasons. Any surgical procedure, particularly of the lower abdominal area, may cause urinary retention. Spinal anesthesia may prevent the client from feeling the urge to void, thus causing urine retention.

A decrease in blood flow (e.g., hemorrhage, shock, hypotension, dehydration) may be manifested by a decrease in urine formation. Early detection of postoperative urinary complications is a major nursing responsibility.

Key interventions and rationales
1. Assess the client for restlessness, agitation, and increased blood pressure.
   These may be signs of a full bladder.

2. Palpate for bladder distention.
   Retention of urine causes the bladder to distend, which may be palpated just above the symphysis pubis.
3. If not contraindicated, let male clients stand to void and have female clients sit on commode or on bedpan in bedside chair.
   Many clients cannot void while lying in bed; a more normal position may induce voiding.
4. If not contraindicated, give the client privacy.
   For some clients, voiding with another person in the room is not possible.
5. Turn on tap water so the client can hear the sound of running water; pour measured amounts of warm water over the perineum.
   These techniques may precipitate voiding. Measuring the water lets you accurately measure the volume of urine voided.
6. Notify health care provider if voiding does not occur 6 or 8 hours after surgery.
   Although every attempt should be made to avoid catheterization, it may be necessary if urinary retention persists.
7. If urinary catheter is in place, monitor for hourly output greater that 30 ml.
   Urine output less than 30 ml/hour may indicate fluid loss or need for increased fluid intake via oral and/or I.V. routes.
8. Notify health care provider if the client voids frequently in small amounts.
   This is indicative of urinary retention with overflow.

CHEMOTHERAPY

Overview

Chemotherapy is the use of drugs to eradicate tumor cells by interfering with their growth and reproduction. One or more antineoplastic agents may be used to treat a client. Chemotherapy may be used alone or in combination with surgery and/or radiation therapy.

Antineoplastic drugs damage normal as well as tumor cells, particularly those cells that grow rapidly, i.e., bone marrow, epithelium, sperm, and hair follicles. These drugs are highly toxic and cause a wide variety of adverse effects, which nurses play a vital role in assessing and managing.

Routes of administration
1. The route of administration for chemotherapeutic agents depends on the drug being administered, the dose, and the neoplasm that is being treated.
2. Chemotherapeutics may be administered topically, orally, intravenously, intramuscularly, subcutaneously, arterially, intracavitarily, and intrathecally.

Adverse effects
1. Antineoplastic drugs are toxic to normal as well as tumor cells and cause many adverse effects.
2. The nurse is responsible for knowing the specific adverse effects for each drug administered.
3. Adverse effects can be grouped by the body system affected:
   - Gastrointestinal system--nausea, vomiting, diarrhea, anorexia, stomatitis, and hepatotoxicity
   - Hematopoietic system--leukopenia, anemia, and thrombocytopenia
   - Renal system--hyperuricemia, hyperkalemia, hyperphosphatemia, hypocalcemia, cystitis (may be hemorrhagic), and renal failure
   - Cardiac system--tachycardia, dysrhythmias, and heart failure
   - Respiratory system--pulmonary fibrosis and pneumonitis
   - Reproductive system (female)--early menopause and permanent sterility
   - Reproductive system (male)--temporary or permanent sterility and sperm mutation
   - Neurologic system--hearing loss, peripheral neuropathies, paralytic ileus, loss of deep tendon reflexes, and confusion
   - Integumentary system--alopecia, rashes, and tissue necrosis (with extravasation of some drugs)

CLASSIFICATION OF CHEMOTHERAPEUTIC AGENTS

Antineoplastic agents are classified according to their action on the reproduction cycle of the cell, either cell-cycle specific (acting on one phase of cell reproduction) or cell-cycle nonspecific (acting independent of the reproductive phases). Within these two headings, they are further classified according to chemical groups. This table lists commonly used drugs by their cellular action.

Cell-cycle specific	Cell-cycle nonspecific
Antimetabolites (interfere with DNA synthesis) cytarabine (Cytosar-U) floxuridine (FUDR) fludarabine (Fludara) fluorouracil (Adrucil, 5-FU) hydroxyurea (Hydrea) mercaptopurine (Purinethol) methotrexate (Folex) thioguanine (6-thioguanine)	**Alkylating agents (cause cross-linking of DNA)** busulfan (Myleran) carboplatin (Paraplatin) carmustine (BCNU) chlorambucil (Leukeran) cisplatin (Platinol) cyclophosphamide (Cytoxan) dacarbazine (DTIC-Dome) ifosfamide (Ifex) mechlorethamine (Mustargen, nitrogen mustard) melphalan (Alkeran) procarbazine (Matulane) thiotepa (Thioplex)
Plant alkaloids (interfere with mitosis) etoposide (VePesid, VP-16) paclitaxel (Taxol) teniposide (Vumon, VM-26) vinblastine (Velban, Velsar) vincristine (Oncovin) vinorelbine (Navelbine)	**Antitumor antibiotics (block synthesis of RNA and DNA)** bleomycin (Blenoxane) dactinomycin (Cosmegen) daunorubicin (Cerubidine) doxorubicin (Adriamycin) idarubicin (Idamycin) mitomycin (Mutamycin) mitoxantrone (Novantrone) plicamycin (Mithracin)
	Hormonal agents (alter cellular growth in tumors that are hormone-sensitive) aminoglutethimide (Cytadren) bicalutamide (Casodex) diethylstilbestrol (DES) estramustine (Emcyt) flutamide (Eulexin) goserelin (Zoladex) leuprolide (Lupron) megestrol (Megace) tamoxifen (Nolvadex) testosterone

Nursing considerations

1. Monitor the client for infection and bleeding.
   Leukopenia (WBC $<6,000/mm^3$) increases likelihood of infection; thrombocytopenia (platelets $<100,000/mm^3$) puts client at risk for bleeding.
2. Monitor the client's vital signs.
   Changes in vital signs may be the first indication of infection in an immunocompromised client.
3. Assess I.V. sites and any areas of skin or mucous membrane breakdown for evidence of infection.
   Open areas may be portals of entry for microorganisms.
4. Observe urine, stools, mucous membranes, and skin breakdown for bleeding. Assess skin for ecchymoses and petechiae.
   Decreased platelets predispose to bleeding.
5. Use meticulous asepsis and handwashing; institute protective isolation if WBC $<1,000/mm^3$; teach the client to avoid crowds and anyone with infections and recent vaccinations.
   This protects client from pathogens in the environment.
6. Teach the client to avoid fresh fruit and vegetables, flowers, and potted plants.
   These items may harbor pathogens.
7. Avoid invasive procedures, i.e., I.V.s, injections, urinary catheters, rectal thermometers, as much as possible. Provide frequent skin care to prevent breakdown. Teach the client to use a soft toothbrush and electric razor.
   Any break in the skin or mucous membranes may be a port of entry for organisms, as well as a site of bleeding.
8. Assess need for stool softener.
   Hard stools may irritate colon, causing bleeding and/or infection.
9. Encourage physical activity, unless contraindicated.
   Decreases the likelihood of skin breakdown and stasis of respiratory secretions, possible sources of infection.

Nutrition

1. Avoid use of commercial mouthwashes.
   Many commercial mouthwashes contain alcohol.
2. If the client develops stomatitis, use an antifungal mouthwash (nystatin [Mycostatin]). An anesthetic mouthwash (lidocaine [Viscous Xylocaine]) may be necessary prior to meals.
   Stomatitis can be very painful, preventing the client from eating properly.

3. Administer antiemetics 30 minutes before meals, if necessary.
   Decreasing nausea/vomiting may make the client amenable to eating.
4. Implement pain-relief measures, as appropriate.
   Pain may cause anorexia.
5. Provide foods high in protein and calories in small, frequent feedings.
   Foods high in nutritional value are necessary for tissue repair. Large amounts of food at one time may cause anorexia. Consider tube feedings or total parenteral nutrition (TPN) if client cannot consume enough food to meet nutritional needs.
6. Assess intake and output (I&O), weight, serum electrolytes (sodium, potassium, chloride, carbon dioxide content), and renal function tests frequently.
   Anorexia, vomiting, and diarrhea may adversely affect the client's fluid and electrolyte balance. Some chemotherapeutic agents are nephrotoxic.

Body image

1. Encourage the client to experiment with wigs, caps, or scarves prior to the onset of alopecia. Explain that all body hair may be affected.
   Being prepared will help the client cope with the alteration in body image caused by hair loss.
2. Be sure that the client understands that the hair will grow back after chemotherapy is over.
   Focusing on the temporary nature of the hair loss will help the client cope with this distressing adverse effect of chemotherapy.

Skin integrity

1. Assess skin daily for rashes, pruritus, jaundice, breakdown.
   Skin disturbances, often accompanied by itching, are common adverse effects of chemotherapy. Hepatic dysfunction may be signaled by jaundice. Areas of skin breakdown are sites for infection and bleeding.
2. Provide antihistamines (lotions and/or systemic) and soothing colloidal baths if the client develops pruritus. Keep fingernails short.
   Itching promotes scratching, which may lead to infection, and also disturbs rest.
3. If the client develops diarrhea, clean anal and perineum with mild

soap, rinse well, and pat dry. Apply medicated ointment, i.e., A and D, if area is excoriated.
Diarrheal fluid is extremely irritating to skin. Excoriation can lead to infection and bleeding.
4. Assess I.V. sites for infiltration, extravasation.
Chemotherapeutic agents can cause necrosis if they get into subcutaneous tissue. Early detection is necessary to minimize tissue damage.

Fatigue
1. Monitor hemoglobin, hematocrit, and erythrocyte counts.
Chemotherapy causes bone marrow depression, with decreased production of RBCs.
2. Assess the client for fatigue, headache, dizziness, and shortness of breath on exertion.
These are indicative of anemia.
3. Help the client plan for frequent rest periods.
This will conserve the client's energy for essential activities of daily living (ADLs).
4. Increase iron and vitamin C in the diet. Use supplements, if the client cannot get enough from food.
Iron will help prevent or mitigate anemia. Vitamin C improves iron absorption and promotes healing and resistance to infection.
5. Administer filgrastim (Neupogen) as prescribed.
This stimulates proliferation and differentiation of hematopoietic cells.
6. Be prepared to transfuse RBCs.
Clients who have severe, symptomatic anemia unresponsive to dietary management and supplements need transfused RBCs to ensure adequate delivery of oxygen to the cells.

Personal protection
1. Chemotherapeutic agents are known to be hazardous to persons handling them. Exposure can occur through direct (skin, mucous membrane) contact with the agent, inhalation, and ingestion.
2. Because of the hazards involved, governmental agencies, nursing organizations, and individual health care agencies have developed guidelines to be followed by those who handle chemotherapeutic agents.
3. The guidelines are:
   a. Prepare chemotherapeutic agents under a laminar flow hood to

prevent inhalation and release into the air.
b. Wear a cuffed gown and latex gloves when handling these drugs, the body fluids of clients receiving chemotherapy, and materials contaminated by their excretions.
c. Make sure all needles, syringes, I.V. equipment, etc., have luer-lock connections.
d. Place a sterile pad over the end of the equipment to collect any of the drug that may be expelled if air bubbles are expelled from syringes and I.V. tubing.
e. Put an absorbent pad under the injection site to absorb any of the drug that spills.
f. Wash skin thoroughly with soap and water if any if the drug comes in contact with it. Eye contact is handled by flushing with copious amounts of water, with the eyelid held back. Examination by a health care provider is necessary after eye contact.
g. Dispose of all equipment in puncture-resistant, leak-proof containers, in accord with regulations governing disposal of biohazardous material. Contaminated linen should be handled using isolation procedures.
h. Wash hands after removing gloves.

RADIATION THERAPY

Overview

Radiation therapy is the use of electromagnetic waves to kill cancer cells in localized lesions by interfering with their growth and reproduction through the disruption of the cells' DNA. It may be used as the sole therapy or combined with surgery and/or chemotherapy. As with chemotherapy, radiation damages normal as well as tumor cells, especially those that divide rapidly. Thus, bone marrow, skin, GI epithelium, sperm, and hair follicles are likely to be destroyed during radiation therapy.

Types of radiation therapy
1. External radiation--the source of the radiation is outside of the body.
2. Internal radiation (brachytherapy)--the radiation source is placed in the body, at the intended delivery site.

METHODS OF DELIVERING RADIATION THERAPY

Several different methods of delivering external and internal radiation exist. This table shows the common delivery methods.

External	Internal
• Kilovoltage--used for superficial lesions of the skin and breast • Gamma ray (cobalt or cesium)--used for lesions below the skin surface • Linear accelerator--used for deeper lesions; tends to decrease skin damage; less scatter of radiation • Cyclotron--used for lesions resistant to other types of radiation therapy	• Needles, seeds, catheters, or wires are used to place the radiation source as close as possible to the cancerous lesion. • Intracavitary--placed in body cavities (e.g., vagina, abdomen) • Interstitial--implanted in involved tissues, either temporarily or permanently

---

Radiation therapy adverse effects

1. Radiation therapy affects rapidly dividing normal cells as well as tumor cells. Many of the adverse effects are the same as those caused by chemotherapy.
2. Because radiation therapy is applied to a localized area of the body, the adverse effects manifested depend on the area being irradiated, i.e., alopecia with radiation to the head; nausea, vomiting, and diarrhea with radiation to the colon.
3. Many clients have systemic adverse effects, such as fatigue, headache, nausea, and vomiting, regardless of the body area being irradiated.
4. Radiation therapy may cause irreversible fibrosis in irradiated tissues. Sometimes, this occurs long after the course of therapy has been completed. If vital organs (i.e., lungs, heart) become fibrotic, the client may experience severe complications, including death.

Nursing considerations

Clients undergoing radiation therapy need to be monitored for infection, bleeding, nutrition, body image, skin integrity, and fatigue, as does the client undergoing chemotherapy. Additionally, the following are specific to clients undergoing radiation therapy.

External radiation

1. Do not remove radiation markers (port marks) from the skin.
   These identify the precise area for irradiation and must remain on the skin.
2. Instruct the client not to use soaps, powders, lotions, cosmetics, perfumes, or ointments on the area being irradiated. Plain water should be used to cleanse the area.
   Some skin products increase radiation dosage and others may further irritate already erythematous skin.
3. Advise the client to keep area protected from excessive heat, cold, and sunlight.
   These may further damage the skin.
4. Tell the client that loose cotton clothing may increase his comfort.
   This lets air circulate and prevents irritation from tight garments.
5. Teach the client to use only an electric razor if the area of irradiation must be shaved.
   Straight-edge razors may irritate and injure to skin made sensitive by radiation.
6. Use care to avoid opening blisters that occur from the radiation.
   Open areas are susceptible to infection.

Internal radiation

Having an implanted radiation source makes the client a radioactive hazard to others until the implant is removed. The following measures should be taken to protect the staff and client.

1. Give the client a private room.
   While internal radiation is in place, other clients must be protected from radiation.
2. Prior to inserting the implant, explain that staff will be limiting the time spent in the room. Help the client plan diversionary activities, i.e., books, television.
   Explanation and interesting activities will help the client feel less isolated.
3. Position the client to maintain integrity of the implant.
   Intracavitary implants (i.e., vaginal, uterine) may be dislodged if the client sits upright or stands.
4. Insert an indwelling catheter if the implant is in the area of the urinary bladder.
   This keeps the bladder empty, increasing its distance from the radiation source.
5. Have the client assume as much self-care as possible. Staff giving

care should do so in as little time as possible and care should be rotated among staff members.

Decreasing exposure time protects staff from radiation.

6. Make sure each care provider wears a dosimeter.

   This device measures total cumulative exposure to radiation.

7. Maintain as much distance from the client as possible, consistent with the need to provide appropriate care.

   Increasing distance from the radiation source protects staff from radiation.

8. Tell anyone who is under 18 years of age, pregnant, or lactating not to visit or care for a client who has internal radiation.

9. Keep an appropriate container (usually lead) in the client's room in case the implant becomes dislodged. Caregivers should wear lead-lined aprons and gloves, if appropriate.

   Shielding protects staff from radiation.

CHAPTER 4

Mental Health Nursing

CRISIS INTERVENTION

Overview

Crisis occurs when one's usual modes of coping no longer work. The precipitating event may be as dramatic as a natural disaster or as ordinary as moving to a new location. Crisis development occurs in the following stages: the precipitating event *(phase 1);* feeling threatened *(phase 2);* usual coping modes fail *(phase 3);* and resolution *(phase 4).*

According to Aguilera's Crisis Model, people who have a *realistic perception of events, adequate social supports* and *adequate coping skills* are not prone to experiencing crisis. The absence of any one of these "balancing factors," however, predisposes the individual to experiencing crisis.

Nurses interact with clients in crisis in a variety of settings, including mental health centers, crisis centers, emergency services, in the community following natural disasters or traumatic experiences such as mass shootings, in office practices, and over the telephone while covering "hotlines." Whatever the setting or circumstance, the nurse must assess and respond to the client's immediate need. If the client is homicidal or suicidal, hospitalization will be required.

The goal of crisis counseling is the restoration of equilibrium. The focus of sessions is the immediate situation and what needs to be done at the moment. Crisis intervention is not a long-term therapy. Clients are expected to regain equilibrium within a short time, usually within 6 weeks. Depending upon the precipitating event, the client's personal strengths and the availability of personal supports, there may be need for a referral for ongoing counseling or support.

Key assessments and rationale

1. Assess what the client views as most problematic or most important at the moment.
   This gives a picture of the situation and a place to begin.
2. Assess the presence or absence of the balancing factors.
   The client will not regain equilibrium until all balancing factors are in place.
3. If the client is involved in a physical trauma such as assault or disaster, assess his physical condition.
   Lower-level needs must be met before higher-level needs emerge.

Attend to the physical first, the psychological second.
4. Assess the client's anxiety level.
Nursing interventions are affected by presenting anxiety level.

Key interventions and rationales
1. Help the client identify some small thing to work on.
This empowers the client and channels his anxiety.
2. Help the client gain a realistic perception of the event, identify available resources, and delineate ways of dealing with the event.
This restores balancing factors and enhances recovery from crisis.
3. Attend to any physical needs.
This demonstrates concern, builds rapport, and frees up energy to work on restoration of balancing factors.
4. Stay with the client or have someone stay with him if needed.
Levels of anxiety may fluctuate rapidly. Depending on the event, the client may feel unsafe and need the security of another's presence.

Consult with the text used in your nursing program for:
NANDA diagnostic statements
Nursing process

ANXIETY DISORDERS

Overview

Anxiety is a common human experience, which--depending on its level--enhances or hinders the client's ability to function. At the *mild* level, anxiety sharpens his perceptual powers and enhances cognitive functioning. At the *moderate* level, anxiety interferes with his ability to function optimally. Perception is somewhat decreased, but problem solving is possible with assistance. Selective inattention allows the client to grasp only certain aspects of an experience, so recall of an event is incomplete.

At the *severe* level, his perceptual field is considerably narrowed so problem solving is very limited along with his ability to be self-directed and responsible for himself. At the *panic* level, problem solving is impossible, safety becomes an issue, reality orientation may be disturbed, and many physiological symptoms will manifest. Clients experiencing either severe or panic level anxiety should be carefully monitored by another and *should not be left alone.* They need a highly structured, calm environment. Safety is a nursing priority.

MANIFESTATIONS OF ANXIETY			
Emotional	**Cognitive**	**Behavioral**	**Physiological**
Lack of spontaneity	Selective inattention	Disorganization	Increased pulse
Irrational fears	Distractibility	Rapid speech	Changes in appetite
Irritability	Distortions in thinking	Inability to relax	Increased blood pressure
Worry	Low concentration	Pacing	Nausea and/or vomiting
Lability			Sweating, dry mouth
			Dilated pupils

Most clients experiencing anxiety disorders are treated on an outpatient basis. It is not uncommon for those experiencing anxiety disorder to concurrently experience clinical depression. With the combination of behavioral therapy and specific medications (selected SSRIs or other antidepressants, or benzodiazepines), most clients with anxiety disorders lead productive lives. Briefly presented below are some of the anxiety disorders nurses commonly observe.

Selected anxiety disorders

Panic disorder: Characterized by sudden and unpredictable attacks of panic level anxiety. Because the first anxiety attack may have happened in a public place, it is not unusual for the client to also develop agoraphobia.

Generalized anxiety disorder (GAD): Characterized by persistent, pervasive anxiety that disrupts the client's quality of life.

Obsessive-compulsive disorder (O/CD): Characterized by irrational thoughts that invade the client's mind unbidden, creating immense anxiety, which is relieved by performing rituals or acts.

Specific phobia: Characterized by irrational fear of something which in reality is harmless.

Posttraumatic stress disorder (PTSD): Characterized by the repeated reliving of a traumatic life event over which the client felt utterly helpless and/or a life event in which he believed death or serious harm was imminent.

Key assessments and rationales
1. Assess the client's anxiety level.
   Nursing interventions are directed by anxiety level.
2. Assess environmental cues that precipitate anxiety.
   This lets the client plan in advance for potentially anxiety-stimulating events.
3. Assess life areas (work, ability to meet daily needs, social life) affected by the anxiety.
   This provides information about the pervasiveness of the anxiety and the need for medication.

Key interventions and rationales
1. Provide for the safety needs of a client whose anxiety level is severe or above.
   Narrowed perceptions make him unable to accurately take in and interpret environmental cues, placing him at risk for self-injury.
2. Teach anticipatory planning to clients experiencing GAD, specific phobia, and PTSD.

This enables the client to plan ahead for potentially anxiety-provoking situations. With such planning, successful management of the situation is increased.

Consult with the text used in your nursing program for:
Names of specific medications
NANDA diagnostic statements
Use of nursing process

COMMONLY USED MEDICATIONS BY TYPE BY ANXIETY DISORDER	
Disorder	**Medication**
GAD	Benzodiazepines (BZDs)
Phobia	Monamine oxidase inhibitors (MAOIs); BZDs
O/CD	Tricyclics (TCAs); SSRIs; Beta blockers
Panic disorder	MAOIs; TCAs; SSRIs; BZDs
PTSD	MAOIs; TCAs; SSRIs

SOMATOFORM DISORDERS
Overview
Clients with somatoform disorders may be preoccupied with body sensations or appearance, or they may demonstrate symptoms without the presence of appropriate underlying pathophysiology. These clients characteristically are treated by primary care physicians who may not recognize the presence of a mental disorder.

Many of these clients have experienced their symptoms for years and seeking treatment is for them an integral part of their lives. As a group, these clients are sincere in their symptom presentation, not realizing the underlying nature of their illnesses. They truly believe that they have "legitimate" physical conditions. Unlike malingerers, clients with somatoform disorders are not deliberately seeking monetary reward or some other advantage (secondary gain) produced by the symptom.

Somatization disorder: Characterized by aches and pains for which the client seeks treatment. He may go to a variety of health care providers seeking relief.

Conversion disorder: Characterized by the presence of sensory or motor symptoms for which no adequate cause is found. The classic example is paralysis of a limb.

Pain disorder: Characterized by the presence of pain (actually perceived/experienced), which is precipitated by psychological needs and disrupts the client's daily functioning. Quality of life is affected.

Hypochondriasis: Characterized by the presence of symptoms, which the client interprets as serious in nature, despite repeated assurances that there is nothing seriously wrong. The person lives in constant fear that health care professionals are "missing" something important and failing to "correctly" diagnose the problem.

Body dysmorphic disorder: Characterized by preoccupation with a body part, which the person judges to be defective and for which correction is sought (e.g., liposuction on a woman who is a size 4 but perceives small deposits of fat on her hips or thighs as ugly).

Key assessments and rationales
1. Physical assessment.
   Whenever there is a physical complaint, underlying pathology must be ruled out.
2. Psychological assessment.
   Many clients with psychosomatic disorders have underlying unmet psychosocial needs.

Key interventions and rationales
1. Perform the examinations required by the symptom presented
   Rule out underlying pathology and prevent lawsuit.
2. Refer to a certified therapist if no underlying pathophysiology supports presenting symptoms
   Unless underlying needs are met, the client will continue to experience physical symptoms. Somatization may be a symptom of depression.

Consult with the text used in your nursing program for:
   NANDA diagnostic statements
   Nursing process

MOOD DISORDERS

Overview

Mood disorders include a range of illnesses from mild depression to bipolar disorder. These disorders are associated with neurotransmitter dysregulation of serotonin, norepinephrine, epinephrine. Also associated with depression is daily length of exposure to natural sunlight. Clients with seasonal affective disorder (SAD) respond positively to exposure to a full-spectrum light during the late fall and winter months, when they tend to experience the "winter doldrums."

The feeling of depression is a common human response to loss. Grieving the loss of a loved one, a pet, a job or social position is expected. Healthy individuals get over these losses in time and continue to carry on despite feeling blue or down. However, depression affects the client's quality of life for an extended time and does not tend to lift without medical intervention. Clinically depressed clients experience significant changes in sleep patterns, eating patterns, self- esteem, energy level, ability to perform both socially and on the job, ability to care for self, and mood.

Since any client who experiences depression is at risk, however small, for suicide, a lethality assessment needs to be completed with initial contact and with each contact thereafter. If in an in-patient setting, clients assessed to be suicidal can be placed on suicide precautions (SP) by the nurse (a physician's order is not needed) until it is deemed the client is no longer suicidal.

Most clients with depression respond positively to a combination of medication and cognitive therapy. Medications commonly used include traditional antidepressants such as the tricyclics, SSRIs, or MAOIs. Dietary restrictions with the MAOIs make their use precarious with clients who cannot or will not adhere to dietary restrictions. Serotonin syndrome is a risk if the client's medication is changed from one classification of antidepressant to another. Thus, a 2-week lag time between dosing from one type of antidepressant to another (e.g., MAOI to SSRI) generally is recommended.

With the antidepressant medications, there is a lag time between the time the medication is started and the beginning of symptom relief. With TCAs and MAOIs, symptom relief may not be noted for up to 6 weeks. With the SSRIs, symptom relief may not be noted for up to 4 weeks. Clients getting these medications need to be educated about this lag time to prevent feeling discouraged. Additionally, the health care provider may need to experiment with medications to discover which one works most effectively with a given client. If this is necessary, the client could be without significant symptom relief for several months.

Clients experiencing bipolar disorder experience at least one episode of depression followed by an episode of acute mania. During an *acute episode of mania,* the client exhibits an expansive/euphoric mood, irritability if constrained in any way, lack of respect for others' boundaries, lack of ability to settle down for sleep, high energy, inability to sit still long enough to eat properly, inattention to personal hygiene, lack of regard for external realities leading to excessive spending or gambling, inflated sense of capabilities ("There is nothing I cannot do") and hypersexuality.

Stabilization of mood is generally accomplished by administering lithium carbonate, which has a narrow therapeutic window. This means that what is therapeutic for one client may be toxic to the next. When taking lithium, the client must maintain adequate fluid and sodium intake to prevent toxicity. Signs of lithium toxicity include severe diarrhea, ataxia, blurred vision, coma, severe vomiting, tinnitus, muscular weakness, marked tremor, lethargy, hyperreflexia, slurred speech, incoordination, seizures, death.

In the event the client cannot tolerate lithium, carbamazepine (Tegretol) or valproic acid (Depakene) may be used to stabilize mood.

Depression
Key assessments
1. Assess the client's suicide potential.
   Suicide is always a risk in a client with depression.
2. Assess the client's mood.
   Depressed mood and anhedonia is characteristic of a depressed client.
3. Assess the client's self-care needs: hygiene, grooming, and nutrition (weight loss or gain).
   Inattention to self-care and changes in weight can indicate presence of depression.
4. Assess the client's sleep pattern and energy level.
   Changes in sleep pattern and lack of energy generally are evident in depressed clients.
5. Assess the client for the presence of worthlessness and/or guilt.

These feelings are present in many depressed clients.
6. Assess the client's thought processes.
Difficulty concentrating and a preoccupation with death are often present.

Key interventions and rationales
1. Ask the client directly if he is suicidal. If he is suicidal or at high risk for suicide, place him on SP.
This maintains the client's safety. He should remain on SP until the nurse is satisfied he no longer is at risk for suicide.
2. Ask the client what he wants to accomplish from treatment.
This communicates the nurse's expectation that the client has a future and that the current situation can change, and it gives the client a goal to work toward. The nurse can assess how realistic the client is about expectations. Unrealistic expectations are a set-up for future failures and resentments.
3. Ask the client what he is willing to do to stay well.
This reveals the client's ability to commit to a treatment plan and reminds him of his responsibility to maintain his health.
4. Teach the client about depression.
The more the client understands about his illness, the better able he will be to deal with it and the more likely he will be to commit to the needed treatment regime.
5. Teach the client about medications.
This enhances adherence to drug therapy. The MAOIs have dietary restrictions that the client must follow or a hypertensive crisis with potential for death can result.

A drug commonly used in this disorder
1. Amitriptyline (Elavil)--this antidepressant inhibits the uptake of serotonin and norepinephrine. Dose range: 75 to 150 mg/day PO. Nursing considerations include monitoring blood pressure and ECG for hypotension and arrhythmias; teaching the client to rise slowly to avoid postural hypotension; cautioning him about driving because of drowsiness as an adverse effect; suggesting sugar-free candy to minimize dry mouth.

Bipolar disorder
Key assessments
1. Assess the client's impulse control and distortions in thought processes.

This provides information about safety needs.
2. Assess the client's response to lithium.
Lithium has a narrow therapeutic window and toxicity can develop quickly.
3. Assess the client's self-care needs: hygiene, grooming, elimination, and nutrition.
This provides information about nursing needs.
4. Assess the client's energy level.
Excess energy puts the client at risk for physiological collapse.
5. Assess fluctuations in the client's mood.
This indicates needs for safety and effectiveness of medication.

Key interventions and rationales
1. During acute manic episode, provide a structured, nonstimulating environment.
The client is hypersensitive to external stimuli during acute manic episode and likely to lose control and either harm self or others.
2. Monitor the client's activities.
An acutely manic client should not be given access to objects that he could use to harm others.
3. Let the client rest or sleep, as he can. Do not worry about a topsy-turvy sleep routine when client is acutely manic.
Exhaustion is a real danger during an acute manic state. Letting the client rest or sleep whenever his body will let him enhances his physiological safety. A regular sleep pattern can be reestablished once the mania is under control.
4. Let the client have a sleeping area away from roommates.
Because the acutely manic client cannot settle down to sleep and will be up roaming about, he should have a sleeping place away from roommates so he does not disturb their sleep.
5. Let the client have finger foods to eat "on the run."
During acute mania, the client may not be able to sit at table to eat. Allowing nutritious finger foods assures adequate caloric intake.
6. When the client's acute mania is under control, teach him about his illness and develop a plan with him for remaining functional in the community.
The more understanding the client has about his illness, the better able he will be to take control of it and the more likely he will adhere to the treatment plan.
7. Teach the client about his medications, especially signs of toxicity and the importance of blood serum monitoring every 3 months.
Knowledge about his medications and their role in controlling his disease will increase adherence. Because the therapeutic window for lithium is narrow, the client needs to know the signs of toxicity

for his own safety and what to do if they appear.
8. Teach the client's family about his illness.
   The vast majority of the mentally ill return to their families after hospitalization. Family members need to understand what they can do for their loved one.
9. Give the client and his family information about the Alliance for the Mentally Ill.
   This group is designed to support secondary consumers of mental health services (families). If the local chapter does not provide support services to families, it will know about the resources available in the client's local area.

A drug commonly used in this disorder
  1. Lithium carbonate (Eskalith)--this mood stabilizer reduces manic behavior by inhibiting the release of neurotransmitters into the synaptic space. Dose range during acute phase 1,800 mg; 300 to 1,200 mg per day in divided doses for maintenance. Nursing considerations include teaching the client the signs of toxicity; telling him to have serum levels of drug measured regularly and to avoid foods with caffeine and high sugar; and warning female clients not to breast-feed while on drug.

Nutrition considerations
  1. Eat high-energy snack-type foods and avoid sugar drinks and caffeine products during manic phase.
  2. Maintain fluid intake of 2,000 to 3,000 ml per day.

TARGET BEHAVIORS AND NURSING INTERVENTIONS WITH CLIENTS EXPERIENCING MOOD DISORDERS	
Depression	**Bipolar disorder, acute manic episode**
Weight loss or gain • Offer small portions of easily swallowed foods q2-3h for weight loss. • Offer low-calorie foods if weight gain present.	**Weight loss** • Have readily available "pick-up" foods that can be eaten "on the run."

TARGET BEHAVIORS AND NURSING INTERVENTIONS
WITH CLIENTS EXPERIENCING MOOD DISORDERS

Depression	Bipolar disorder, acute manic episode
Sleep pattern disturbance (insomnia) • Instruct the client to get out of bed. • Offer warm milk and crackers. • Teach relaxation techniques. • Eliminate any distracting stimuli. • Allow for quiet music if soothing. • Teach about sleep disturbance as part of the illness.	**Sleep pattern disturbance (hyperactive)** • Establish a bedtime routine. • Allow catnapping to prevent physiological collapse. • Place in a private area at night. • Avoid caffeine. • Avoid stimulating activities after the evening meal.
Self-care deficits • Assist with self-care as needed. • Accompany to meals and assist with food selection. • Monitor elimination patterns.	**Self-care deficits** • Supervise self-care activities to assure appropriate presentation of self. • Do not require client to sit down to eat.
Guilt • Listen to expressions of guilt. • Ask client what needs to happen for self-forgiveness to occur. • Help the client use the cognitive technique of reframing.	**Irritability** • Observe for pattern. • Allow for alternative choices when limits must be set. • Avoid caffeine.
Dependency • Do not require decision making when energy is low. • Acknowledge lack of energy and teach about this as being a part of the disease. • State expectation that the client will eventually care for self. • Help the client do small tasks for self.	**Hyperactivity** • Provide a nonstimulating environment. • Provide structured, large muscle activity. • Keep presentation of self calm. • Keep number of choices to a minimum.
Constipation • Increase fluid and bulk in diet. • Get an order for a prn laxative. • Make the client move around (walk, do activities).	**Impulsivity** • Be aware of safety issues. • Monitor spending and sexual activity. • If the client is irritable, keep at least an arm's length and a leg's length away from him.
Low self-esteem • Provide accomplishable tasks. • Be attentive to self-care needs. • Spend time with the client. • Use compliments sparingly. • Do *not* be overly cheerful.	**Emotional lability** • Redirect behavior. • Do not take behavior personally. • Maintain a calm, detached manner.

<table>
<tr><td colspan="2" align="center">TARGET BEHAVIORS AND NURSING INTERVENTIONS
WITH CLIENTS EXPERIENCING MOOD DISORDERS</td></tr>
<tr><td>Depression</td><td>Bipolar disorder, acute manic episode</td></tr>
<tr>
<td>Somatic complaints
• Give prn meds as appropriate.
• Thoroughly assess each complaint.
• Instruct the client to keep a diary of complaints.</td>
<td>Disruptive, loud behavior
• Remove client to a quiet area.
• Redirect into a structured activity.
• Use a quiet, calm tone of voice.
• Do not match the client's volume level or affect.</td>
</tr>
<tr>
<td>Internalized anger
• Require client to participate in a daily routine to externalize pooled energy. Enjoyment is not the issue; neither is liking or wanting.
• Use large muscle activity such as walking or kneading bread.</td>
<td>Delusions of grandeur
• Do not directly challenge the delusion.
• Redirect the client into a reality-based activity.</td>
</tr>
<tr>
<td>Self-berating
• Do not forbid expression.
• Redirect into an accomplishable task.</td>
<td>Social inappropriateness
• Provide 1:1 supervision as needed.
• Tell the client in simple, clear language what is acceptable.
• Model appropriate behavior.</td>
</tr>
<tr>
<td>Boredom/fatigue
• Provide diversions.
• Make the client attend activities.</td>
<td>Refusal to take medications
• Provide with written material about the medication.
• Give choices--"Do you prefer liquid or pill form?" "Do you prefer to take medicine now or in 10 minutes?"</td>
</tr>
</table>

Consult with the text used in your nursing program for:
Medications
NANDA diagnostic statements
Nursing process

SCHIZOPHRENIA

Overview
Schizophrenia is considered a disease of the brain. An excess of the neurotransmitter dopamine as well as structural changes in the brain are associated with this disorder. Clients with this disorder face many challenges induced by such negative symptoms as anhedonia, avolition, poverty of speech, blunting of affect, poor grooming, poor

attention span, and apathy. Although the some symptoms of schizophrenia such as bizarre behavior, agitation, loose associations, hallucinations, and delusions respond to medications, adhering to a medication regime has proven difficult for many clients. Relapse is common following discontinuance of medication.

Socially, many clients with schizophrenia find sustaining ongoing relationships problematic and do not tolerate high levels of stress. This intolerance makes full-time employment as well as close living with others difficult.

Key assessments and rationales
1. Assess the areas of the client's life that are affected.
   The ability to meet the demands of daily living contributes the quality of life and the ability to live independently.
2. Assess the client's thought processes.
   Disturbances in thought processes interfere with the client's ability to meet the demands of daily living. Thought disturbances may further interfere with his ability to reliably adhere to a prescribed medication regime.
3. Assess the client for presence of hallucinations and length of time he has experienced hallucinations.
   Clients who have hallucinated for years will most likely not be totally free of hallucinations but can be taught techniques for controlling them. Failure to control hallucinations interferes with ability to function optimally.
4. Assess the client for adherence to medication regime.
   Consistency in dosing is a major factor in controlling the positive symptoms of schizophrenia and letting the client live in the community.
5. Assess the client for job skills.
   The ability to support himself contributes to the client's positive self-esteem and lessens social withdrawal.

Key interventions and rationales
1. Provide assistance as needed for life-skills management. Life skills include ability to dress and groom appropriately, negotiate transportation, secure and prepare food, maintain a living space, meet one's own needs for affiliation, pursue a fulfilling activity, and maintain a balanced life-style.
   Such assistance lets the client perform optimally.
2. Provide the client with a structured routine.

Predictability reduces stress, which can contribute to social isolation, hallucinatory activity, and delusions.

3. Give the client tools for controlling hallucinations and/or, if in an in-patient setting, distract him as soon as hallucinatory activity is evident.

   Control of hallucinations is important if the client is to function in the community. Hallucinatory activity is exhausting and leaves limited energy for reality-based activity.

4. Give the client mechanisms for medication adherence. For example, clients who cannot remember to dose daily might be good candidates for a depot medication.

   Adherence to medication regime enhances control of symptoms that interfere with ability to function adequately. For clients who resist medication, changing to the atypical antipsychotics such as resperdal, clozaril, or zyprexa may be helpful.

5. Refer the client for occupational evaluation.

   Participation in gainful activity, even for a few hours a day or week, can do much to "mainstream" the client into the larger social order, decreasing the negative effects of social withdrawal and enhance self-esteem.

Target behaviors and nursing interventions with schizophrenic clients	
Altered thought processes (delusions, illogical actions, disorganization)	• Provide a structured environment. • Never directly challenge a delusion. Ask about it and seek clarification. Respond to the message of the delusion. • Engage the client in a reality-based activity. • Limit the number of caregivers per shift.
Sensory-perceptual alteration (hallucinations)	• Provide a structured environment. • Ask about the hallucination to understand what he is experiencing. • Redirect the client to reality-based activities. • Teach the client techniques for interrupting hallucinatory activity (e.g., humming, listening to another person). • Observe for when hallucinations occur and plan accordingly. • Intervene the moment you suspect the client is beginning to hallucinate.
Impaired verbal communication (loose associations, neologisms)	• Respond to any themes you can identify. • Ask the client what he wants you to understand. • Ask the client what he means.

Target behaviors and nursing interventions with schizophrenic clients	
Impaired social interaction	• Honor space requirements. • Do not bombard the client with verbiage. • Engage the client in a nonthreatening activity. • Spend prearranged time with the client to build trust. • Limit the number of caregivers per shift. • Keep emotional expressiveness low.
Self-care deficits	• Supervise the client's self-care. • Give the client structure by having written instructions available. • Establish a self-care routine. • Give positive reinforcement for desired changes.
Sleep-pattern disturbances	• Establish a bedtime routine. • No caffeine after 4 p.m. • No napping after 2 p.m. • Provide soothing activity 2 hours before bedtime. • Eliminate distracting environmental stimuli.
Nonadherence with medication regime	• Determine if the client has a preferred medication. • Give the client choices about how/when to take the medication (e.g., depot vs daily dosing, dosing schedule). • Assess any adverse effects and intervene vigorously. • Teach the client about the importance of taking medication to control the mental illness. • Discuss symptom management with the client.
Fluid volume excess (water intoxication)	• Monitor the client's fluid intake. • Check specific gravity. • Monitor the client's behavioral symptoms. • Teach the client about the dangers of water intoxication. • Teach the client how to monitor own intake.

Consult with the text used in your nursing program for:
Medications
Dosing
Major adverse effects especially agranulocytosis, neuroleptic
    malignant syndrome, dystonia, and tardive dyskinesia
    (clozapine and risperidone have been known to reverse this
    otherwise irreversible adverse effect).
Nursing measures

GOALS FOR CLIENTS WITH SCHIZOPHRENIA

- Depending on severity of illness and compliance with medication, the client may be able to assume major responsibility for own grooming and self-care and may be able to hold a limited job and care for own living space.

- For clients who have had schizophrenia for years, the external structures need to remain as functional as possible. For example, the client will need reminders to take medication and attend day-care because of his inability to sort through confusing stimuli.

- Clients severely affected by schizophrenia will need someone to provide verbal and physical assistance with basic tasks such as hygiene, meal preparation, and care of living space.

A drug commonly used in this disorder

1. Haloperidol (Haldol)--this antipsychotic blocks the uptake of dopamine. Dose range: 0.5 to 5 mg, two to three times a day. Nursing considerations include teaching the client and family about adverse effects and their management which is important for increasing adherence to medication.

SUBSTANCE-RELATED DISORDERS: SUBSTANCE ABUSE/CHEMICAL DEPENDENCE

Overview

Generally speaking, chemical dependence follows a predictable pattern, beginning with experimentation and ending with dependence. For those who become dependent on their substance(s) of choice, the only way of controlling intake is abstinence. Additionally, many clients find it necessary to join a support group such as Alcoholics Anonymous (AA); Narcotics Anonymous (NA) or Cocaine Anonymous (CA) to maintain an abstinent life-style.

Chemical dependence is strongly associated with family history, so completing a three-generation genogram is helpful when taking an initial substance use history. Careful exploration of the effects of substance use on the client's life provides a comprehensive picture for determining abuse. Life areas to be explored are depicted in the table below.

LIFE AREA	WHAT TO EXPLORE
Spiritual	Violations of ethical or moral values--e.g., lying, cheating, stealing
Physical	Deterioration in health--e.g., hangovers, hypertension, gastritis, esophageal varicosities
Mental	Impaired judgment while under the influence; blackouts
Emotional	Embarrassment, guilt, defensiveness about one's consumption, use of defense mechanisms (denial, rationalization, minimization), personality changes
Family	Broken promises, feeling nagged by members to stop or cut down, family members making excuses for the user's behavior
Social	Loss of friends, increasing amounts of time spent pursuing the substance to the exclusion of relationships, bar-mates become one's "buddies"
Leisure	Abandonment of formerly pleasurable hobbies or activities
Economic	Debt because increasing amounts of money spent on the substance(s) of choice
Sexual	Impotence, careless or risky sexual behavior during blackouts or while under the influence
Legal	Traffic violations, bar fights, domestic violence
Vocational	Absenteeism because of hangovers or pursuit of the drug, decline in quality of work or productivity, inability to hold a job

Key assessments and rationales

1. Assess the client's physical condition.
   Many clients have substance-induced or related medical conditions requiring treatment. Considering Maslow's hierarchy of needs, lower-level needs must be met before higher-level needs can emerge. Depending on the substance abused, signs of withdrawal need to be identified and appropriate action taken, especially for withdrawal from alcohol.
2. Assess the client's substance use.
   This provides information about potential for withdrawal syndrome and magnitude of the problem.
3. Assess the client's perception of the situation.
   Work with the client's perceptions, not the nurse's.
4. Assess what areas of the client's life are affected.
   This indicates how pervasive the effects of substance use are on the client's life.
5. Assess the client's coping skills.
   Use/abuse of substances is associated with poor coping/ stress management skills.
6. Assess the client's willingness to limit use or adopt an abstinent life-style.
   This provides information about the client's potential for adhering to a treatment program.

Key interventions and rationales

1. Attend to any physical symptoms and engage in the appropriate withdrawal protocol.
   Prevent complications from withdrawal and other medical conditions. Following the protocol for alcohol withdrawal is crucial to prevent delirium tremens (DTs), coma, or death.
2. Use appropriate screening instruments such as the CAGE for alcohol use.
   Using an appropriate screening instrument enhances nonjudgmental data collection, decreasing defensiveness.
3. Ask the client what he hopes to gain from treatment.
   This provides information about the client's readiness for treatment.
4. Ask the client specifically about the life areas depicted in the table above.
   This will help raise the client's consciousness about effects of substance abuse in his life. Once consciousness has been raised, the client will become more willing to consider life changes.

5. Ask the client to list coping skills and rate the effectiveness of each one. Ask about the use of specific substances to relieve stress.
This will help the client become consciously aware of his coping skills and their effectiveness. If coping skills are limited or ineffective, he can learn new ones or fine-tune or discard old ones.

6. Educate the client about the effects of the substance on his body and in his life.
Knowledge is power. Knowing how his physical, mental, emotional, and social well-being is affected by substance abuse can help the client make a conscious decision to change. Educating him about the biologic factors associated with substance abuse can help him take a more objective look at the effects of substance use in his life.

7. Give the client a list of resources, introduce him to an appropriate support group, and help him get a sponsor.
Developing an adequate support system is important for maintaining abstinence. Associating with others who are in recovery gives the client a perspective that he cannot get on his own. It also provides others from whom he can draw support. Recovery is a lifelong process requiring on-going work, including networking with others.

CAGE QUESTIONNAIRE TO IDENTIFY ALCOHOL ABUSE

1. Have you ever felt you should cut down on your drinking?

2. Have people annoyed you by criticizing your drinking?

3. Have you ever felt bad about your drinking?

4. Have you ever had a drink in the morning to steady your nerves or get rid of a hangover?

Two affirmative responses indicate addiction.

Drugs commonly used in this disorder

1. Disulfiram (Antabuse)--this alcoholic deterrent interferes with the metabolism of alcohol. Dose range: 125 to 500 mg/day. Nursing considerations include monitoring for signs of disulfiram reaction (sweating, headaches, violent vomiting, confusion, and respiratory depression); and teaching the client to not use alcohol while on the

drug and to take the drug when going to bed to avoid daytime sedative effect.

2. Naltrexone (Re Via)--this narcotic antagonist blocks the effects of opium derivative ingestion. Dose range: 25 to 50 mg/day. Nursing considerations include monitoring for overdose of opioids; teaching the client to not use alcohol or opiates while on medication; and emphasizing not to take OTC drugs because they may contain small amounts of opiates.

Consult with the text used in your nursing program for:
Signs of intoxication, withdrawal, and nursing care by substance
NANDA diagnostic statements
Use of nursing process
Detoxification procedures
Medications used in early recovery

EATING DISORDERS:
ANOREXIA NERVOSA AND BULIMIA NERVOSA

Overview

There is a preoccupation with thinness among many women in affluent nations. This preoccupation has led to the development of eating disorders that generally first manifest in adolescence and, for many, continue over a lifetime. Although men can develop eating disorders, 90% of people with anorexia nervosa or bulimia nervosa are women. Thus, these disorders are considered to be a woman's disease. Although there is research associating eating disorder with neurotransmitter imbalance and evidence that eating disorder runs in families, there is still much that is unknown.

Most of the women who develop either of these disorders are preoccupied with the shape of their bodies and equate success and acceptability with thinness. The woman with anorexia nervosa does not view her eating pattern as abnormal. Refeeding is difficult because of her distorted body image and irrational fear of losing control and getting fat.

On the other hand, the woman with bulimia nervosa is more difficult to identify because she is often within normal weight range. It is the dentist who may first identify the woman with bulimia nervosa because of enamel erosion on the inner surfaces of her teeth. The woman with bulimia nervosa is embarrassed about her compulsive binging and purging behavior. Following a binge, she may feel depressed and be at risk for suicide. She may be relieved when someone asks her about her behavior and be more receptive to treatment than her anorexic counterpart.

Both groups of women are in danger of dying from their disorder; the anorectic woman from malnutrition and the bulimic woman from electrolyte imbalance. Both groups of women may exercise to excess as a means of burning calories.

Key assessments and rationales
1. Assess the client's physical health.
   This is to determine the progression of the disease. Pay special attention to height, weight, body temperature, blood pressure, hair, skin, nails, neurological functioning, and peripheral vascular system.
2. Assess the client's perception of her body size.
   The greater the distortion of body image, the harder it will be to engage this woman in treatment.
3. Assess the client's self-expectations.
   Many women with eating disorders strive for unrealistic perfectionism.
4. Assess the client's social skills.
   Many women with eating disorders have strained relationships because of control issues.

Key interventions and rationales
1. Obtain lab values and ECG.
   This provides data about cellular functioning
2. Monitor the client's food intake and activity level.
   Especially for the woman who restricts her intake, minimal calorie requirements need to be met to attain a medically safe weight. Frequent small feedings will be more acceptable to this client than three meals a day. A bowl of cottage cheese or a supplement such as Ensure will create less anxiety for her than a bowl of ice cream. Exercise must be carefully monitored to conserve energy for weight gain.

3. Help the client establish healthy goals and realistic expectations for meeting these goals.
   Because of an intense need for perfectionism, the client will benefit from learning how to set realistic performance expectations. Asking her how a given action will accomplish her goal or prove her competence is one way to challenge her self-expectations in a relatively nonthreatening manner.
4. Enroll the client in a group for women with eating disorders.
   Developing an alliance with others who have similar needs and fears instills hope and decreases the sense that no one understands and that one is all alone. In the safety of the group, the client can explore the pros and cons of maintaining her eating pattern and experiment with alternatives.

Consult with the text used in your nursing program for:
   Medications used with individuals with eating disorders
   NANDA diagnostic statements
   Implementation of the nursing process

Drugs commonly used in this disorder
1. An antianxiety agent may be prescribed. There are no specific drugs to reverse or cure anorexia nervosa.

Nutrition considerations
1. A calibrated diet that gradually increases weight at a target rate. Rapid weight gain is unsound and dangerous because of potential cardiovascular overload.

CRITICAL THINKING EXERCISE

Mental Health Nursing

Facts and objectives
1. The NCLEX-RN tests your ability to make sound clinical judgments.
2. Developing critical thinking skills is the foundation for being able to make good clinical judgments.
3. This exercise will help you evaluate how well you think critically.
4. As you work through this exercise, you will learn how the continuous flow of questions that evolve as you think the case through will lead you to reach solid conclusions about the client problem and the *best* nursing behaviors.

Instructions
Respond to the following questions by writing down your best thoughts, ideas, and "answers" in the space provided. Do this for all of the questions, then turn the page to see what you should have considered in response to each question.

Naturally, to learn to think critically, don't look for hints or answers before completing all questions...don't cheat yourself! How you answer the critical questions will depend on how well you perfect your thinking skills.

1. How would the nurse determine if the client was experiencing a crisis or an anxiety disorder?

2. What distinguishes a grieving person from a person with clinical depression?

3. What distinguishes panic disorder from PTSD?

4. How would the nurse determine if a client was exhibiting agranulocytosis or acute flu?

5. Someone experiencing acute mania and someone experiencing clinical depression both exhibit self-care deficits. How do the nursing interventions differ?

6. A client believes that his food is being poisoned. What is the best way to respond without reinforcing the delusion and at the same time planting seeds of doubt?

7. In her case load, the case manager has a client who has long-term schizophrenia. This client does not take his medications as directed and does not show up for clinic visits. What would be the best actions for the case manager to take to improve adherence?

8. What criteria would the nurse use to determine if the client was at risk for withdrawal syndrome from alcohol?

9. A client with anorexia nervosa was admitted to an in-patient unit because of low weight (85 pounds, 5"10"). Refed to 98 pounds, she has been told that she can leave the hospital once she reaches 100 pounds. The nurse enters her room to weigh her in the morning at the usual time. The client's weight is 100 pounds (the day before it was 98). The client expresses her delight and asks the nurse to start the discharge process. What should the nurse do?

THE FOLLOWING ARE INTERVENTIONS AND NURSING BEHAVIORS YOU SHOULD HAVE CONSIDERED IN ANSWERING THE PREVIOUS QUESTIONS.

1. How would the nurse determine if the client was experiencing a crisis or an anxiety disorder?
• *In a crisis, there generally is an identifiable precipitating event. Although there is an aspect of loss and a balancing factor may be absent, the crisis is a turning point for growth, and the client may feel ready to change. The client may have limited life experience, but in most cases there is no comorbid psychopathologies.*
• *With an anxiety disorder, the cause may be unclear or unknown. There may be a biological component, and the client may have a genetic predisposition (in many cases, there is a positive family history). The client's anxiety might not be reality-based and may be associated with comorbid depression; he may require medication for relief.*

2. What distinguishes a grieving person from a person with clinical depression?
• *A grieving person won't feel any loss of self-esteem and will be able to complete self-care activities. Felt in response to a specific loss, grief will resolve on its own.*
• *A clinically depressed person will feel guilty, hopeless, and despairing, have low self-esteem, possibly be self-loathing. Depression does not generally resolve without intervention and may include a biologic or genetic component.*

3. What distinguishes panic disorder from PTSD?
• *Panic disorder is unpredictable attacks of anxiety with no specific cause. In most cases, sleep is not disturbed.*
• *PTSD is precipitated by a traumatic event, causes severe sleep disturbances, and includes flashbacks.*

4. How would the nurse determine if a client was exhibiting agranulocytosis or acute flu?
See if the client is taking a neuroleptic and if his WBC is below normal.

5. Someone experiencing acute mania and someone experiencing clinical depression both exhibit self-care deficits. How do the nursing interventions differ?
• *Supply clients experiencing acute mania with finger foods, eliminate distractions in the environment interfering with ability to complete self-care, and monitor appropriateness of dress.*
• *Select foods for clients experiencing clinical depression and feed them if necessary, make them attend meals, monitor them for constipation, and bathe them if they're too fatigued to do for themselves. Also, select their clothing if they're too fatigued.*

6. A client believes that his food is being poisoned. What is the best way to respond without reinforcing the delusion and at the same time planting seeds of doubt?
Ask the client what evidence he has about his food being poisoned. If the client says that the kitchen workers are spies placed in the hospital to poison him, express wonderment about how

people on the unit are not showing any signs of poisoning. Ask him how he thinks that might be. Reflect back to him any messages that are reflected in his speech. For example, the message might have something to do with needing to feel safe. The nurse might "wonder" if the client is feeling unsafe on the unit and further ask what would make the client feel safe. After having determined the essence of the client's message and responding to it, the nurse should redirect the client into a reality-based activity.

7. In her case load, the case manager has a client who has long-term schizophrenia. This client does not take his medications as directed and does not show up for clinic visits. What would be the best actions for the case manager to take to improve adherence?
First, the case manager needs to assess why the client is not reliable about taking his medications. If memory impairment is the problem, she may need to call the client at dosing time to remind him to take the medication or stop by his place to medicate him. If adverse effects are the problem, the case manager needs to negotiate what will be acceptable to the client and work with him, the pharmacist, and the health care provider to find a medication acceptable to the client. If transportation to the clinic is the problem, it needs to be arranged. The more the client can be included in the care plan, the greater the chance that he will adhere to it.

8. What criteria would the nurse use to determine if the client was at risk for withdrawal syndrome from alcohol?
The nurse would get a history of previous withdrawal syndrome, review the history of abuse (length of time of abuse, tolerance level, stage of addiction), find out when the client last had a drink, and monitor the client's pulse, pupils (dilated), diaphoresis, tremor, and restlessness. If any of these signs are positive without other causes, the nurse would suspect withdrawal and initiate a detoxification protocol.

9. A client with anorexia nervosa was admitted to an in-patient unit because of low weight (85 pounds, 5"10"). Refed to 98 pounds, she has been told that she can leave the hospital once she reaches 100 pounds. The nurse enters her room to weigh her in the morning at the usual time. The client's weight is 100 pounds (the day before it was 98). The client expresses her delight and asks the nurse to start the discharge process. What should the nurse do?
First of all, this client's weight gain probably is not valid. The nurse should tell her that she will record the weight and consult with the health care provider. About 2 hours later, she should return to the client's room with a gown, ask the client to put it on and tell her that she needs to reweigh her to validate the weight. Many clients "hold" urine in their bladder to add weight, or they cleverly attach weights to their clothing. To discharge this client without reasonable assurance that the weight is valid would contribute to her demise.

Maternity Nursing

ANTEPARTAL CARE

Overview

The time from conception to the beginning of labor is the antepartal period. The focus of nursing care in this period is to maintain health and prevent pregnancy complications for the client and her developing fetus. The nurse engages in many roles while interacting with the client and her family to ensure optimal outcome for physiological, psychological, and sociocultural adaptations to pregnancy.

Normal adaptations to pregnancy

Antepartal care begins with establishing the client's baseline history and current physical and emotional status. This includes assessing her family and social support in her environment.

Initial history assessment

- General health history (assessing for pre-existing health conditions that will create a high-risk pregnancy, such as diabetes, cardiac disease, renal disease, etc.)
- Family health history (any genetically transmitted diseases in the family)
- Menstrual history (determine age of onset, last menstrual period, expected date of delivery, any complications)
- Obstetrical history (gravida, para, abortion, GTPAL)
- Occupational history (conditions in the work environment that affect pregnancy)
- Religious/cultural background

Physiological changes of pregnancy

1. Reproductive system
   - Uterine enlargement (hypertrophy) begins in response to elevated estrogen. There is also an increase in the number of cells (hyperplasia). The uterus rises to the symphysis pubis by the 12th week, umbilicus by 20th week, and xiphoid process by the 38th week; lightening occurs by the 40th week. There is a marked increase in the amount of blood flow to the uterus.
   - Vaginal changes in response to estrogen result in increased vascularization and hypertrophy. The vaginal secretions are thick, white and acidic. This environment is more susceptible to yeast infections.
   - Cervical changes in response to estrogen cause mucous plug (operculum) development; the increased vascularity causes a

bluish discoloration (Chadwick's sign) and softening of the cervix (Goodell's sign).
- Ovulation ceases; the corpus luteum continues the production of hormones, especially progesterone to maintain the pregnancy.
- Breasts increase in size and the areola darkens. Colostrum secretion may begin in the third trimester.

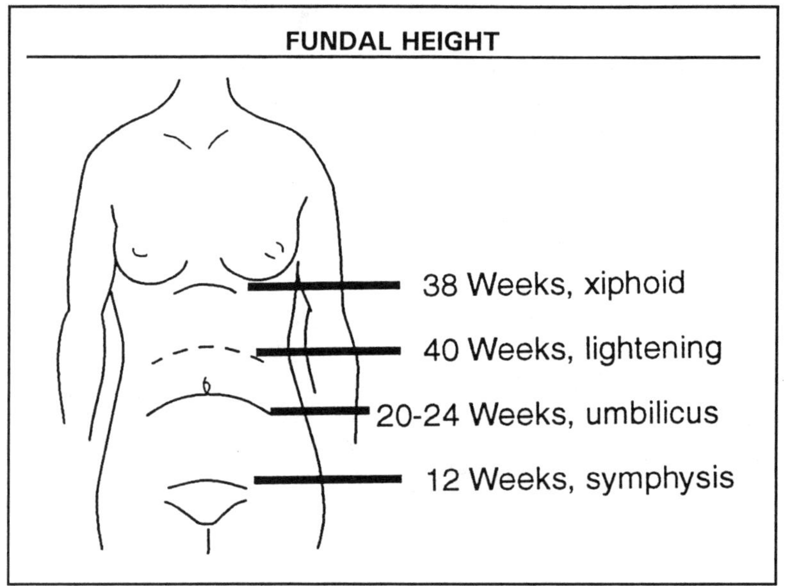

2. Endocrine system
   - Slight enlargement of the anterior pituitary gland. Prolactin is secreted to support lactation. Posterior pituitary stimulates oxytocin production for uterine contractility and milk ejection.
   - Thyroid increases in size, producing more thyroxine, increasing basal metabolism rate (BMR) and causing some heat intolerance.

3. Respiratory system
   - Diaphragm moves upward and the anteroposterior diameter enlarges. Slight increase in respiratory rate and slight hyperventilation occurs.
   - Vascular changes result in common complaints of respiratory congestion, epistaxis, and earaches.

4. Cardiovascular system
   - The heart is displaced up and slightly to the left. Hypertrophy occurs because of increased blood volume and cardiac output. Heart rate increases by 10 to 15 beats per minute (bpm) by term. Blood pressure drops slightly in the second trimester and returns to baseline by the third.
   - Blood volume increases by 40%, two-thirds being plasma volume and one-third being RBCs, causing pseudo anemia.
   - Cardiac output increases from 30% to 50%. WBCs increase to $12,000/mm^3$ by term, increasing to $25,000\ mm^3$ during labor.
   - Increases in fibrin, plasma fibrinogen, and coagulation produce a hypercoagulable state during pregnancy and early postpartum.

5. Renal system
   - Kidneys enlarge slightly and the ureters dilate. Glomerular filtration rate and blood flow to the kidneys increases by 50%.
   - Increased pressure on the bladder occurs during the first and third trimester from the gravid uterus.
   - Urinary stasis leads to increased risk of infection.
   - Glucosuria may appear during pregnancy and indicates the need for further testing for gestational diabetes.

6. Gastrointestinal system
   - Progesterone causes a decrease in gastrointestinal tone and motility.
   - There is an increased sensitivity to taste and smell.
   - Nausea and vomiting are common in the first trimester because of elevated human chorionic gonadotropin (hCG) levels.
   - Ptyalism (excessive salivation) and gingivitis (inflammation of the gums) may be apparent.
   - Constipation and hemorrhoids can occur because of decreased motility, increased water absorption, and pressure from the gravid uterus.
   - Gallbladder function is decreased and can lead to hypercholesterolemia, predisposing the woman to gallstone formation.
   - Typically, women gain 25 to 35 pounds during pregnancy.

7. Musculoskeletal system
   - The hormones progesterone and relaxin cause softening and

stretching of the uterine supportive ligaments, which support the gravid uterus.
  - The center of gravity changes as weight of pregnancy increases, causing a responsive lordosis.
  - Diastasis recti of the abdominal muscles may occur at the linea alba in the midline as they separate from the enlarging uterus.
  - Calcium intake needs to be sufficient to prevent demineralization of the maternal skeleton.

8. Integumentary system
  - Increases in estrogen and progesterone result in hyperpigmentation of the skin.
  - Striae gravidarum (stretch marks), spider nevi, linea nigra (darkened line from the umbilicus to the pubic area), darkened nipples and areola, chloasma (or melasma, the "mask of pregnancy"), increased nail growth, and palmar erythema are all skin changes that may occur in a normal pregnancy.
  - The generalized feeling of warmth is a result of increased blood flow to the skin.

9. Hormone changes
  - Human chorionic gonadotropin (hCG) is secreted by the trophoblast in early pregnancy to stimulate progesterone and estrogen production. This is what positive pregnancy tests are based on.
  - Human placental lactogen (hPL or human chorionic somatomammotropin), an insulin antagonist, decreases maternal metabolism of glucose that is needed for the developing fetus.
  - Estrogen is secreted by the corpus luteum and then the placenta. It stimulates uterine development of the fetus.
  - Progesterone, produced by the corpus luteum and then the placenta, is considered "the hormone of pregnancy." It inhibits uterine contractility and maintains the endometrium.
  - Relaxin is secreted by the corpus luteum and in small amounts by the placenta. It aids in the effects of remodeling collagen and softening of the cervix.

10. Psychosocial changes
  - The first trimester is characterized by a state of ambivalence. The client needs anticipatory guidance, support, and validation

as she accepts the task of pregnancy.

- The second trimester is characterized by the reality of fetal movement and definition. The mother fantasizes about the identity of the fetus and the motherhood role. The client needs support and education about the physical changes her body is experiencing.
- The third trimester is characterized by concern over the birth process and bringing a baby into the world.
- The nurse needs to provide continued support and education through childbirth classes and home preparation after birth.

Key assessments and rationales

1. Do initial head-to-toe exam to establish baseline data.
   - *An elevated blood pressure warrants follow-up for pregnancy-induced hypertension (PIH). Elevated temperature may mean infection.*
   - *Weight gain should be 25 to 35 pounds total. Pelvic measurements: Diagonal conjugate at least 11.5 cm. Obstetrical conjugate is estimated.*
2. Identify presumptive, probable, and positive indicators of pregnancy.
   - *Presumptive changes are subjective in nature. They include amenorrhea, nausea and vomiting, fatigue, urinary frequency, breast changes, and quickening.*
   - *Probable changes are objective. They include Chadwick's sign, Hegar's sign, uterine enlargement, and positive pregnancy test.*
   - *Positive signs of pregnancy are fetal heart rate and fetal movement.*
3. Assess the client's learning needs.
   Identify educational level and best mechanism to teach the client.

Key interventions and rationales

1. Instruct the client on the danger signs of pregnancy, which she should report immediately.
   Vaginal bleeding could indicate threatened abortion, placenta previa or abruption. Gush of fluid could indicate a premature rupture of membranes. Persistent vomiting could be hyperemesis gravidarum. Chills and fever could be infection. Abdominal pain could be an ectopic pregnancy or abruptio. Visual disturbances, severe headache, and swelling of the face and hands is indicative of PIH.
2. Direct the client to take medications only approved by her health

care provider.

Prescription and nonprescription medications can be harmful to the fetus, particularly during weeks 2 to 8, the period of fetal organogenesis. This includes consumption of tobacco, alcohol, and illicit drugs.

3. Teach the client how to minimize morning sickness.

   She should eat small, frequent, high-protein meals, and avoid spicy and fried foods. Crackers before arising from bed in the morning may be helpful. She will have an increased sensitivity to smells.

4. Outline future antepartal visits.

   Monthly visits through 32 weeks gestation, bimonthly through 36 weeks gestation, and then weekly until delivery. Prenatal care is important for the best outcome of pregnancy. If a high-risk problem occurs, visits will need to become more frequent.

5. Encourage exercise and safety precautions.

   Walking is the best exercise if the client had no previous exercise routine. The client's center of balance has changed, and she is at increased risk of injury. Minimize height of heels on shoes. Advise her to wear supportive comfortable clothing.

6. Teach the client to maintain good hygiene habits.

   The client may take baths or showers in pregnancy, unless a high-risk condition occurs. She can continue with routine dental care and should be shielded if x-rayed. Douching is contraindicated in pregnancy. No immunizations with live virus should be given. The client should ambulate every 2 hours when on extensive trips or at work to maintain good peripheral circulation.

7. Discuss sexual activities during pregnancy.

   The client may continue with sexual intercourse during pregnancy. She needs to communicate with her partner about comfort and position changes. Sexual intercourse is contraindicated if there is vaginal bleeding, fluid leaking, or contractions. If these occur, the client needs immediate follow-up with her health care provider.

8. Teach preventive measures for the discomforts of pregnancy.

   - *For constipation and hemorrhoids: adequate fluids, fruits and vegetables, and regular exercise.*
   - *For leg cramps: elevate legs and dorsiflex feet.*
   - *For backaches: pelvic rocking and back massage with counter-pressure.*

9. Prepare the client for the birth process.

   Prepared childbirth classes are usually attended in the third trimester. These classes provide an expanded knowledge base and teach coping techniques for the childbirth experience. They focus on breathing and distraction techniques to improve the birth experience.

10. Teach the client warning signs of impending labor.
    Lightening, urinary frequency, weight loss, bloody show, spurt of energy, and membrane ruptures are premonitory signs of labor.

Drugs commonly used during antepartum

1. Most antepartal clients will be on prenatal vitamins during pregnancy. Many clients also take an iron supplement t.i.d. Prenatal vitamins and iron supplements help provide the increased amounts necessary for a healthy pregnancy.

Nutritional considerations

1. There is an increased need for all nutrients during pregnancy. A well-balanced diet is essential for proper development of the fetus. (See nutrition table)

NUTRITIONAL NEEDS OF PREGNANCY

Nutrient	NonPregnant	Pregnant	Nutrient used for	Recommended foods
Protein	60 g	76 to 100 g	Fetal tissue growth Placental growth and development Maternal uterus and breast growth Increased maternal circulating blood volume, hemoglobin and plasma protein Storage reserves	Milk, grains, cheese, eggs, legumes, nuts, meat
Calories	2,100	2,400	Increased energy	Carbohydrates, fats, proteins
Minerals Calcium	800 mg	1,200 mg	Fetal bone formation Fetal dental enamel forming cells Maternal calcium metabolism	Cheese, eggs, whole grains, leafy vegetables
Phosphorus	800 mg	1,200 mg	Fetal tooth formation Increased maternal metabolism	Milk, cheese, lean meats
Iron	18 mg	18+mg and 30 to 60 mg supplement	Increased maternal circulating blood volume High iron metabolism during pregnancy	Whole grains, eggs, liver, beans, nuts, leafy vegetables
Iodine	100 mcg	125 mcg	Increased metabolic rate Increased thyroxine production	Iodized salt
Magnesium	300 mg	450 mg	Protein metabolism Tissue and cell metabolism Muscle function	Soybeans, cocoa, whole grains, dried beans, seafood
Vitamins A	4,000 IU	5,000 IU	Cell and tissue growth Fetal tooth and bone formation	Butter, cream, margarine, green & yellow vegetables

NUTRITIONAL NEEDS OF PREGNANCY

C (ascorbic acid)	60 mg	70 mg	Tissue formation and integrity Cement in connective and vascular tissues Increased iron absorption	Citrus fruits, berries, tomatoes, melons, chili peppers, green vegetables
Thiamine	1 mg	1.3 mg	Coenzyme in energy metabolism	Pork, liver, beef, beans
B12	3 mcg	4 mcg	Coenzyme in protein metabolism, especially vital cell proteins, such as nucleic acid	Milk, eggs, meats, liver, cheese
Folic acid	400 mcg	800 mcg and 200 to 400 mcg supplement	Increased pregnancy metabolism Increased hemoglobin production Production of cell nucleus material Prevent neural tube defects	Liver, leafy vegetables

PROBLEMS OF PREGNANCY

Threatened abortion

Overview

Threatened abortion may occur in a client who is at less than 20 weeks gestation. This client manifests vaginal bleeding, cramping, and a closed cervix. This pregnancy may continue if intervention is successful.

Pathophysiology

The causes of a threatened abortion could be formational errors in the product of conception, maternal or fetal infection, hormonal imbalance, and abnormalities of the reproductive system. This differs from an inevitable abortion in which the cervix is dilated and the pregnancy cannot be maintained.

Key assessments and rationales

1. Assess the client's vital signs frequently.
   Look for increased pulse or decreased blood pressure, indicating shock. An increased temperature indicates infection.
2. Assess the client for vaginal bleeding and cramping.

Increased bleeding and cramping may indicate the cervix is dilating. The amount of bleeding may lead to impending shock.

Key interventions and rationales

1. Maintain bed rest and start a pad count.
   Increased activity can lead to increased cramping and possible cervical dilation. There should not be more than one pad/hour saturation.
2. Keep the client NPO and start I.V. fluids.
   The client should be NPO initially until bleeding is stabilized and I.V. fluids (typically lactated Ringer's solution) are initiated to maintain hydration.
3. Order initial lab work for baseline data.
   A CBC, blood type, and screen should be done. If any tissue is passed, it should be sent to the laboratory.
4. Explain all procedures to the client and provide emotional support.
   * *The client will be extremely anxious about this unexpected episode in her pregnancy.*
   * *When cramping and bleeding stop, she will be sent home with restrictions, possibly including bedrest.*

Pregnancy-induced hypertension

Overview

Pregnancy-induced hypertension (PIH) is a common complication of pregnancy that may occur after 20 weeks gestation. The classic triad of symptoms are hypertension, proteinuria, and edema. PIH is further classified by preeclampsia, eclampsia, and the HELLP syndrome. There is an increased incidence of PIH in clients who are primigravida; multiple gestation; are under 16 or over 35; are of African-American heritage; have diabetes, renal disease, or hydatidiform mole; and are of lower socioeconomic status. PIH can contribute to intrauterine fetal death and perinatal mortality.

Pathophysiology

The cause of PIH is unknown. It is based on a number of theories:

1. The maternal cardiovascular, hematologic, and renal systems have maladaptations during pregnancy.
2. There is hemoconcentration instead of hemodilution and plasma volume expansion. The increased blood viscosity to organ perfusion responds by vasoconstriction, resulting in increased systemic vascular resistance and hypertension.
3. This results in increased cardiac output and arterial spasms. The result is a multiple organ system challenge.

Key assessments and rationales

1. Assess the client's vital signs, particularly noting any blood pressure changes.
   The blood pressure is diagnostic. If the systolic level has increased 30 mm Hg and/or the diastolic has increased 15 mm Hg from client's baseline, there should be two readings at a minimum of a 6-hour interval for diagnosis. If there is no baseline blood pressure available, a blood pressure of 140/90 indicates hypertension.

2. Assess the client's urinary output and for proteinuria.
   Proteinuria is diagnosed as 1+ (300 mg/liter) or 2+ (1g/liter). Increased proteinuria indicates a worsening of the disease process. Normal urine output should be at least 30 ml/hour or 400 to 500 ml/24 hours.

3. Assess the client for edema and weigh her daily.
   Edema of the hands and feet can be a normal finding in pregnancy. Facial edema is more indicative of PIH. Weight should be done daily on arising every morning; a 3 pounds/24 hours or 4 pounds/3 days indicates PIH.

4. Assess neurological status, deep tendon reflexes, and presence of clonus.
   Altered level of consciousness and visual disturbances result from vasospasms. The client may present with scotomata, blurred vision, or headache. Deep tendon reflexes should be 2+. Hyperreflexia and presence of clonus indicate progression of the disease.

5. Assess the client's respiratory status.
   Decreased respirations, dyspnea, and crackles indicate progression of the disease.

Key interventions and rationales

1. Teach the client signs and symptoms to watch for that indicate progression of PIH.
   If the client has blurred vision, increased blood pressure, nausea and vomiting, epigastric pain, difficulty breathing, decreased urinary output, or hematuria, she should immediately seek medical intervention.

2. Keep the client in a quiet and well-monitored environment.
   Stress exacerbates this condition. The client needs to be constantly monitored for progression of symptoms. In a hospital environment, the client should be close to the nurse's station and, ideally, in a private room.

3. Encourage side-lying positioning, particularly left side lying. *Side-lying position aids in peripheral vascular circulation and minimizes vena cava compression.*
4. Institute seizure precautions. *Seizures can occur if the client progresses to an eclamptic state. Have padded side rails, suction, and oxygen available.*
5. Initiate fetal monitoring. *If the client is being monitored at home, use kick chart or home modem transmission. In the hospital, a fetal monitor strip should be done every shift and prn.*
6. Provide emotional support for the client and her family. *Fear does not improve this condition. The client needs to be reassured she is in the best setting for her condition. PIH will end 48 hours after delivery.*

Drugs commonly used in this disorder
1. Magnesium sulfate is a CNS depressant that is given to clients to reduce the risk of seizures. As a secondary response of the drug, blood pressure is reduced because of relaxation of smooth muscles. Dose range: 6 g bolus over a 30-minute period as a loading dose; maintenance infusion of 2 to 3 g/hour. Nursing considerations include monitoring level of consciousness, blood pressure, serum magnesium levels (4 to 8 mg/dl), respiratory rate ($>$ 12/minutes), patellar reflex (1+ or higher), clonus, urinary output, and fetal heart tones (FHT) (120 to 160 bpm). Calcium gluconate (1 g I.V. over 3 minutes) is the drug antagonist for magnesium sulfate and should readily be available. This drug is absolutely contraindicated in a client with myasthenia gravis. Monitor carefully any client who has heart block or myocardial damage.

Nutritional considerations
1. A diet high in protein and moderate sodium restriction. (See section on "Low-sodium foods.") Foods high in protein are milk, cheese, eggs, meats, grains, legumes, and nuts.

Gestational diabetes mellitus

Overview

Gestational diabetes mellitus (GDM) has its onset or is first diagnosed during pregnancy. Women who are predisposed to GDM have previously delivered a macrosomic infant, had unexplained fetal loss, maternal obesity, or previous GDM. All pregnant clients are typically screened for GDM between weeks 24 to 28 gestation. A 50 g non-fasting glucose tolerance test resulting in ≥140 mg/dl requires further testing. The goal is to provide an equilibrium in glucose utilization and insulin availability. Women diagnosed with GDM require health education and frequent monitoring as the pregnancy progresses.

Pathophysiology

GDM is a carbohydrate metabolism disorder of varying severity. Diet therapy is initially used to manage the disease, but insulin may be required as the pregnancy progresses. This disease usually resolves in early postpartum. It may recur later in the woman's life as type 2 diabetes mellitus.

Key assessments and rationales

1. Assess the client's blood glucose levels.
   If the 50 g glucose test was >140 mg/dl, a 3-hour glucose tolerance test (GTT) is done. Two or more elevated values are indicative of GDM. Home glucose monitoring consists of q.i.d. testing. Fasting ranges of blood glucose are to be maintained at 60 to 90 mg/dl, and 2-hour post prandial, at 100 to 140 mg/dl. Urine testing is done at all prenatal visits.
2. Assess the client's vital signs, weight gain, and fundal height.
   Elevated blood pressure may indicate PIH. One pound a week weight gain is suggested in the second and third trimester. An increased fundal height could indicate polyhydramnios.
3. Assess the client for signs and symptoms of urinary tract or vaginal infections.
   Glucosuria and urinary stasis provide an ideal environment for development of infection. There is an increased incidence of vaginal yeast infections in these clients.
4. Assess fetal status.
   FHT should remain 120 to 160 bpm. A non-stress test (NST) and oxytocin challenge test (OCT) may be ordered as pregnancy progresses. This fetus is at an increased risk of being large for gestational age (LGA) resulting in cephalopelvic disproportion (CPD) problems. This client may also have an amniocentesis. The results expected would be: 3:1 L/S ratio, presence of phosphatidyl glycerol, positive Nile blue test, decreased bilirubin level, increased creatinine level, and gross appearance of intrauterine debris.

Key interventions and rationales

1. Monitor results of diagnostic tests.

Insulin will have to be increased as pregnancy progresses because of production of human placental lactogen (hPL), which reduces insulin's effectiveness.

2. Teach the client about her disease and self-care.
   Determine the client's knowledge of her disease and her current self-care habits. Review hypoglycemic reactions and metabolic acidosis. Dietary needs will be regulated as pregnancy progresses. She needs to maintain a basic exercise plan and can begin with walking if she's had no previous plan.
3. Schedule follow-up visits.
   This high-risk client should be seen every 2 weeks during early pregnancy and weekly after the 7th month of pregnancy.

Drugs commonly used in this disorder

1. Insulin (see "Pharmacology review"). GDM clients typically require regular and long-acting insulin during the day.
2. Oral hypoglycemics are never used during pregnancy.

Nutritional considerations

1. The client will be on a diabetic diet. The calories will be divided up among three meals and three snacks. To prevent hypoglycemia at night, the bedtime snack must consist of protein and complex carbohydrates. A nutritionist should see this client for proper nutrition teaching. The client will need to familiarize herself with food exchanges for meal planning.

Preterm labor

Overview

Preterm labor is the leading perinatal and neonatal problem today. Maternal, placental, or fetal factors can be the contributing cause. Maternal factors may be pre-existing disease conditions, infection, abdominal surgery, and uterine or cervical anomalies. Placental factors may be abruptio or placenta previa. Fetal factors could be infection, hydramnios, or multiple gestation. The goal of care is to prevent or stop preterm labor from advancing to a delivery state.

Pathophysiology

Labor that begins between 20 and 37 weeks gestation is preterm labor. After the cervix has dilated more than 4 cm and effaced more than 50%, treatment for preterm labor has limited success. The longer the birth can be delayed safely, the better the neonate's outcome.

Key assessments and rationales

1. Assess the client's risk for preterm labor.

Clients who have a previous history of preterm birth, multiple pregnancy, low socioeconomic factor, or poor antepartal care are at risk, as are those who smoke or use cocaine.
2. Assess the client for contractions and cervical changes.
Contractions of any type should be noted. Differentiate if they are Braxton-Hicks, low, dull backache, abdominal cramping without diarrhea, or mild menstrual-like cramps. An increase in vaginal discharge warrants a vaginal exam to check for cervical effacement and dilation.
3. Assess the client's home and work environment activities.
The client should eliminate lifting heavy objects, including children. She should limit pushing and pulling activities and take frequent rests, particularly lying on her left side. She may need to stop work.

Key interventions and rationales
1. Instruct the client on signs of preterm labor.
Teach the client to palpate contractions with her fingertips on the fundus. If they occur every 10 minutes for an hour or if she has rupture of membranes, she needs to seek medical intervention immediately.
2. Teach the client to force fluids.
The client should have 2 or 3 quarts of fluids per day but she should avoid caffeine. Dehydration can initiate preterm labor.
3. Minimize or eliminate sexual activity.
If contractions or rupture of membranes occur, sexual activity is contraindicated. Also, nipple stimulation may illicit uterine contractility.
4. Teach the client coping mechanisms and provide support.
The client will be anxious and needs emotional support and techniques to minimize stress.
5. Encourage bladder emptying.
The client should void every 2 hours while awake.

Drugs commonly used in this disorder
1. Tocolytic drugs are used in the treatment of preterm labor. They suppress or cease contractions and prolong pregnancy. Tocolytics are contraindicated in clients with severe PIH, chorioamnionitis, fetal death, or acute fetal distress. Clients begin with I.V. tocolytic therapy and progress to PO. The most common tocolytics are:
    a. Magnesium sulfate, which is used in women with cardiopulmonary disease, diabetes, or infection. This drug works as a smooth muscle relaxant on the uterus. (Dosage and

adverse effects are covered under PIH, page 110.)
  b. Terbutaline is the most widely used tocolytic. It is a β-mimetic. A maternal adverse effect can be pulmonary edema.
  c. Ritodrine (Yutopar) is a β-mimetic. It is more expensive than terbutaline and used less frequently.
2. Betamethasone--this glucocorticoid is given to a woman in preterm labor to aid in inducing pulmonary maturation and to minimize respiratory distress to the preterm newborn. The dosage is 12 mg once a day for 2 days, given intramuscularly.

COMPARING PLACENTA PREVIA AND ABRUPTIO PLACENTAE

	Placenta previa	Abruptio placentae
Type	*Total:* Placenta lies over the cervial opening. *Partial:* Placenta covers only part of the cervical opening *Marginal:* Low implantation near the cervical opening	*Total:* Premature separation of the placenta from the uterine wall (with total, the separation is complete) *Partial:* Partly separated from the uterine wall
Clinical signs	Painless bleeding in third trimester; signs of hemorrhage; signs of fetal distress; predisposing factor--multiparity in older women; intermittent bleeding	*Total:* Concealed (hidden) or apparent hemorrhage Painful bleeding in third trimester; board-like abdomen (with shock or fetal distress); predisposing factors--preeclampsia, eclampsia, multiparity, and endocrine imbalances; complication--hypofibrinogenemia
Treatment	Hospitalization; bed rest; diagnosis by sonogram. *Total:* With frank bleeding, delivery always by cesarean section *Partial:* Delivery usually by cesarean section *Marginal:* Delivery occasionally by cesarean section	Replacement of blood loss; I.V. fluids; vaginal delivery if possible, cesarean delivery if vaginal not possible
Nursing considerations	Do not perform a pelvic examination; explain procedure to the client; monitor maternal and fetal condition; prepare the client for delivery.	Explain procedure to the client; monitor maternal and fetal condition; prepare the client for delivery.

**VIEW THE PROGRAM *"FETAL HEART MONITORING"*
BEFORE PROCEEDING. IT IS THE 4TH PROGRAM ON
THE VIDEO MODULE.**

INTRAPARTAL CARE

Overview
Intrapartal care begins when the client has her first true labor
contractions and proceeds through birth and the first few hours of
postpartum. The nurse's primary role is educating the client about the
labor process, assessing for labor progress and high-risk conditions,
and providing emotional support for her and her family.

Physiological changes
Labor should begin between weeks 38 and 42 of gestation. There are
many theories about what causes labor. The woman and fetus go
through many physiological adaptations as they progress through the
intrapartal phase. These are:

Maternal changes
1. Premonitory signs that labor is beginning are lightening, Braxton-
   Hicks contractions, bloody show, bursts of energy, and rupture of
   membranes.
2. Regular, frequent uterine contractions--frequency, duration, and
   intensity of contractions is noted.
3. Rupture of fetal membranes--FHT are taken immediately after
   rupture of membranes. Assess color of amniotic fluid and amount.
4. Cervical dilation--cervix dilates from 0 to 10 and becomes 100%
   effaced. A bloody show will appear as cervical dilation occurs.
   The client should not push until the cervix is dilated to 10 or she
   will have cervical edema.
5. Vaginal lesions--any lesions, including herpes, may warrant a
   Cesarean section.
6. Abdominal scars--a previous Cesarean section or abdominal
   surgery may warrant another Cesarean section.

MONITORING UTERINE CONTRACTIONS

Characteristics of uterine contractions
1. Rhythmic--increment, acme, decrement
2. Intermittent--work phase, rest phase
3. Involuntary--no conscious control

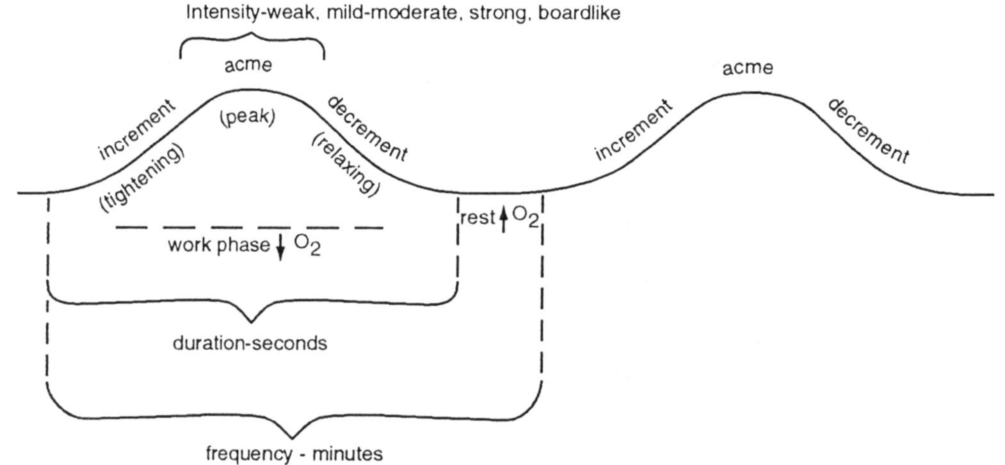

Contraction	Duration	Frequency	Intensity	Cervical changes*
TRUE	Lasts longer as labor progresses	Occurs more often as labor progresses	Become stronger as labor progresses	Effacement; dilation
FALSE	Varies	Irregular	Varies	No significant changes

*Main difference between true and false labor contractions is that false labor contractions tend to diminish when client is ambulating.

Stages of labor

Stage	Contraction characteristics	Maternal physical changes	Fetal position changes
I. Dilation--*Starts with first true labor contraction and ends with complete cervical effacement and dilation* **Phases** • **Early** (latent inactive): *Cervix efaces, dilates 1 to 4 cm; longest, least uncomfortable phase* • **Active**: *Cervix dilates 4 to 8 cm* • **Transitional**: *Cervix dilates 8 to 10 cm; shortest, most uncomfortable phase*	See contraction characteristics for individual phases below • Every 5 to 10 minutes for 20 to 40 seconds • Mild to moderate, increasing in frequency, duration, and intensity • Every 3 to 5 minutes for 40 to 45 seconds • Moderate to strong • Most effacement and dilation in shortest period • Every 2 to 5 minutes for 45 to 60 seconds • Increase in strength and duration; may decrease in frequency	• Percent of effacement • Dilation (1 to 10)	• Engagement • Descent • Flexion • Internal rotation
II. Expulsion--*Starts with complete cervical effacement and dilation and ends with delivery*	• Strong • Upper part of uterus is active; lower part is passive	• Perineal bulging • Crowning of fetal head • Delivery of fetus	• Extension • External rotation • Expulsion
III. Placental stage-- *Starts with delivery of baby and ends with delivery of placenta and membranes*	• Strong • Every 3 minutes	• Placental separation 5 minutes after delivery • Gush of blood • Descent of umbilical cord • Uterus rises in the abdomen and becomes globular • Placental expulsion	

IV. First hour post delivery	N/A	N/A	• Uterus contracted and usually located near umbilicus • Lochia present • Perineum intact

Fetal changes

1. Fetal heart rate--this should remain at 120 to 160 bpm during the labor and birth process.
2. Fetal attitude--the relationship of fetal parts to one another, for engagement and descent through the birth canal (occiput, vertex, bregma, sinciput, face, mentum).
3. Fetal lie--the relationship of the long axis of the fetus to the long axis of the mother (cephalic, breech, transverse).
4. Fetal position--the relationship of the presenting part to the mother's pelvis (ROA, ROP, LOA, LOP).
5. Fetal station--the relationship of the presenting part in relation to the mother's ischial spines (0 is equal with the ischial spines; the more positive the number, the closer the presenting part is to the perineum).

Key assessments with rationales

1. Review the client's prenatal record, including all laboratory tests data.
   This will identify any risk criteria and provide information needed for birth preparation
2. Assess current labor status, including contractions, rupture of membranes, cervical effacement and dilation, last meal eaten, nausea and vomiting.
   This provides data on the client's current stage of labor. Last food intake must be known in case a Cesarean section is needed.
3. Assess the client's preparation for the childbirth experience. Determine if she attended childbirth classes. Is there a support person available? What are her expectations of labor?
   Knowledge of what to expect and having support ease the labor process.
4. Assess the client's emotional state.

This will provide data so appropriate teaching can be done during and after birth process.

Key interventions with rationales
1. Encourage the client to void every 2 hours.
   A full bladder can be uncomfortable and impede delivery.
2. Assist the client with breathing techniques and provide comfort measures.
   Slow, even breathing is best. Avoid hyperventilation. Utilize positioning and distraction techniques to provide comfort.
3. Perform vaginal examinations, as needed.
   This monitors the progress of labor. After rupture of membranes has occurred, this is kept to a minimum.
4. Prepare the client for delivery at the end of the transition phase.
   At the end of transition, there is an increase in bloody show, an urge to push, perineal and rectal bulging, crowning, and uncontrollable leg shaking. The client is now ready for delivery.
5. Position the client for delivery.
   An upright position works best with contractions and best supports the client.
6. Coach the client with her breathing.
   Encourage the client to pant or blow when the fetal head is delivered. This allows for suctioning of newborn, and minimizes lacerations and episiotomy by controlling the expulsion.
7. Praise and encourage the client to see and touch the infant.
   Promotes early attachment behaviors.

PROBLEMS OF LABOR
Dystocia and cesarean section delivery
Overview

Dystocia is a difficult or prolonged labor caused by uterine malfunction or anomaly, fetal size, position, or inadequate pelvic measurements. The presence of any of these factors warrant a Cesarean section delivery.

Pathophysiology

Hypotonic uterine contractions occur when contractions become weak and ineffective, then stop. Pelvic diameter is reduced from contractures or soft tissue abnormality. Stress-released hormones increase anxiety, which can inhibit cervical dilation.

Key assessments and rationales

1. Assess abnormal labor pattern.
   The client presents with slowed or stagnate cervical dilation. There is delay in fetal descent. Frequently there are hypertonic or hypotonic contractions with minimal cervical changes. Abnormal FHT patterns may be present.
2. Assess when membranes ruptured.
   24 hours after rupture of membranes (ROM), there is an increased incidence of infection. Meconium-stained amniotic fluid typically indicates fetal distress.
3. Assess hydration.
   The client should be kept NPO, with a running I.V. to maintain hydration.

Key interventions and rationales

1. Prepare the client for ultrasound.
   Ultrasound will be performed to assess for CPD.
2. Initiate preoperative care for a Cesarean section.
   The client will need an informed consent signed, abdominal-perineal prep, indwelling Foley catheter, and preoperative medication, if ordered.
3. Provide emotional support for the client and her family.
   This is a high stress period for the client and her family. Reassurance and answers to questions are needed and wanted.

Postoperative

1. Provide routine postoperative care.
   Recognizing any postoperative complications early is important. The client is at an increased risk of hemorrhage because of surgery.
2. Perform a postpartal assessment. Assess breasts, fundus, abdominal incision, lochia, and Homan's sign.
   This provides routine postpartal care.
3. Monitor for signs of infection.
   Temperature above 100.4° F after 24 hours, foul-smelling lochia, or pain are early signs of infection.
4. Maintain pain-relief measures.
   Incisional pain can be relieved with analgesics. Discomfort from flatus can be obtained by early ambulation and prone positioning.

POSTPARTAL CARE

Overview

Postpartal care begins after the infant's birth and continues until 6 weeks after delivery. This is a time for the maternal body to return to a homeostatic state after all the adaptations it had made during pregnancy.

Physiological changes

1. Reproductive changes
   - Uterine involution occurs as the fundus (top of the uterus) rises slightly above the umbilicus after delivery and then descends 1 fingerbreath per day. The uterus should remain firm and in a midline position. Usually by 10 days it can no longer be palpated because it returns to a pelvic organ. Exfoliation occurs at the placental detachment site. Lochia is the vaginal discharge that occurs for about 21 days. Lochia rubra is dark red and occurs until day 3. Lochia serosa is lighter in amount and light pink in color, occurring until day 10. Lochia alba is light white-yellow and can occur until day 21. The cervical os closes completely by the first week. Vaginal edema and ecchymosis diminish within 1 week. Suture line healing is complete and vaginal rugae return by 3 weeks. Non-breast-feeding women usually return to menstruation by 6 weeks. Breast-feeding women vary, but menstruation usually occurs by 28 weeks.

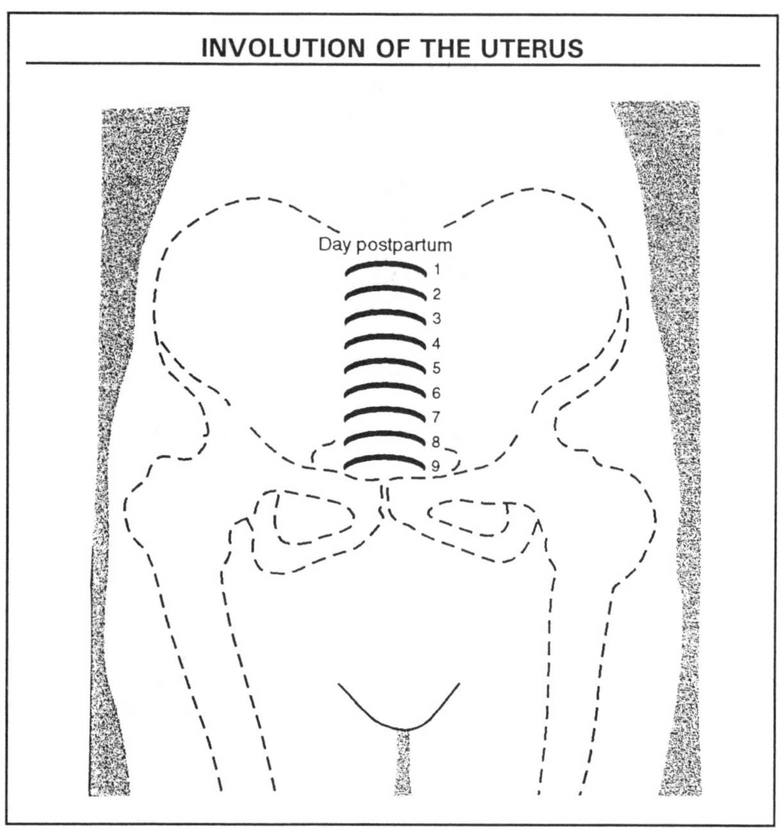

2. GI system changes
   - Hunger and thirst usually are apparent immediately after delivery.
   - GI motility usually remains sluggish for 3 or 4 days.
   - Diastasis recti may be apparent in abdominal muscles. This may return over time with exercise. Striae may be apparent on the skin and fade to a silver color but not completely diminish. Initial weight loss after delivery is 10 to 12 pounds, taking at least 6 weeks to loose the complete 25- to 35-pound weight gain of pregnancy.
3. Urinary system changes
   - The first 12 to 24 hours, the client will have a postpartal diuresis, voiding 2,000 to 3,000 ml.
   - There is occasional hematuria from bladder trauma. Clients are

at an increased risk for developing urinary infection because of dilated ureters and urinary stasis for 6 weeks.

Key assessments with rationales

1. Assess vital signs every 15 minutes for the first 2 hours after delivery.
   Decreased blood pressure may indicate shock. Increased blood pressure could indicate PIH. Pulse will typically be bradycardic the first 6 to 10 days after delivery. Temperature can be up to 100.4° F for the first 24 hours because of stress of labor and dehydration. After that, it indicates infection.

2. Do a complete postpartum physical assessment.
   Perineal checks need to be done every 15 minutes the first hour, then every shift and prn. Breasts will progress from soft, filling to engorged. Nipples should be intact with increased pigmentation and colostrum excretion. Fundus should be firm and in the midline with progressive descent. A boggy fundus requires immediate intervention and massage. Lochia is moderate, becoming progressively scant. Perineum is intact with possible edema or ecchymosis. Hemorrhoids may be present. Homan's sign is negative, bilaterally.

3. Assess attachment behaviors.
   Initially, the client may be quiet and passive from the delivery effort. At 24 to 48 hours, the client should assume responsibility for newborn care, hold en face, identify characteristics, and call infant by name. Identifying "baby blues" versus postpartum depression early on is important.

4. Review laboratory tests.
   Hemoglobin should not be less than 2 g/dl below admission value. WBC range may go as high as 25,000 and is not an indicator of infection. If the client is Rh negative and newborn is Rh positive with negative Coombs', mother will be candidate for RhoGAM. If rubella titer was not immune, she needs to be immunized in postpartum. Urinalysis should be normal; hematuria may be present from lochia contamination.

Key interventions with rationales

1. Teach the client breast and perineal care.
   Encourage her to wear good supporting bra. If an area of the breast gets red and hot to touch, inform health care provider. This may be mastitis. Clients should perform perineal hygiene and change pads after each voiding or defecation to minimize perineal infection. Foul odor from lochia indicates infection.

2. Implement pain-control measures.
   For non-breast-feeding mothers, bind breasts and apply ice. Engorged nursing mothers should be encouraged to nurse more frequently. For episiotomy and laceration discomfort, use ice for 24 hours, sitz baths after first 24 hours. Prescribed topical applications such as pads with witch hazel, analgesic sprays, and analgesia often give relief.
3. Teach the client self-care management.
   The client may take showers or baths. If taking tub baths during the first week, she should be sure to use clean water. The cervix remains open. She may begin gradual exercise, as directed by her health care provider. Ambulate soon after delivery with assistance. Sexual activity may resume when lochia has ceased and the perineum has healed. Review contraceptive options.
4. Encourage optimum rest and sleep.
   Assist the client in plans to incorporate rest and sleep into her schedule, particularly early in postpartum course.

Breast-feeding

Overview
Breast-feeding should begin immediately after delivery. Breast-feeding provides the newborn with an immunological advantage of IgA, which has antiviral and antibacterial properties. Breast milk has a nutritional advantage for newborns. It is more easily digested and absorbed than formula. Breast-feeding is contraindicated in a client with breast cancer, acquired immunodeficiency syndrome (AIDS), or active chemical dependency.

Physiology
Estrogen and progesterone drop in production after birth, leading to increased prolactin production. Prolactin promotes milk production. The infant's sucking action stimulates the release of oxytocin, which stimulates the let-down reflex and increases contractility of the myometrium. This fosters a quicker uterine involution for breast-feeding women.

Key assessment and rationales
1. Assess the client's ability to breast-feed.
   The client needs to be awake and alert to begin the breast-feeding process. Breast-feeding should be culturally and socially acceptable to her. Identify any pre-existing history or medication use that would contraindicate breast-feeding.
2. Assess the client's knowledge and preparation for breast-feeding.
   Assess the client's knowledge of nipple care. Do not use soap on

nipples for bathing; keep them open to air for healing. Use lanolin cream, if prescribed.

Key interventions and rationales
1. Provide privacy and instruction for breast-feeding.
   Discuss positioning; side-lying, sitting, or football hold. Squeeze a small amount of colostrum out and have infant latch on to nipple and areola. The infant probably will suck about 10 minutes on each breast. Break nipple suction with your finger prior to removing infant. Whichever breast the infant finishes on is the breast it will begin on for next feeding. Burp infant in between switching breasts. Infant will breast-feed every 2 or 3 hours.
2. Provide measures to encourage let-down reflex.
   A warm shower, warm drink, plenty of rest, and adequate fluid and protein intake facilitate let-down reflex.
3. Facilitate follow-up on the client's success with breast-feeding after discharge.
   LaLeche or lactation consultants can help the client with successful attempts at breast-feeding, if needed.

Newborn care

NORMAL NEWBORN ASSESSMENT	
Every newborn should have a physical assessment withing 24 hours of birth. This assessment provides baseline data and detect any abnormalities early.	
Assessment	**Normal findings**
1. Check vital signs and blood pressure.	Apical pulse, 120 to 140 bpm; respirations, regular at 30 to 60/minute; audible blood pressure using Doppler device, 70-40 mm/Hg
2. Measure weight, length, head and chest circumference.	Weight, depending on sex: 1,500 to 4,000 g (5 lb, 8 oz to 8 lb, 13 oz); length, 45 to 55 cm (18 to 22 inches); head, 32 to 37 cm (12.5 to 14.5 inches); chest, 30 to 35 cm (12 to 14 inches)
3. Inspect head and fontanels, noting placement of eyes, nose, mouth, and lips.	Face should be symmetrical; no discharge from orifices; pupils equal, reacting to light; patent nose and mouth.
4. Assess skin for color, birthmarks, and intactness.	Should be smooth, no jaundice and with normal hair distribution.
5. Observe chest and abdomen.	Chest should be cylindrical with equal rise and fall. Nipples symmetrical and may be engorged. Abdomen may protrude.
6. Check umbilical cord.	Cord should be trivasular with no bleeding or odor.
7. Inspect buttocks and anus.	Buttocks should be symmetrical, folds separated by a crease. Anus is patent with meconium passing within 24 hours.
8. Evaluate limbs for flexion, symmetry, adduction and abduction, and muscle tone.	Will try to assume fetal position. Should be full range of motion with no asymmetry.
9. Assess genitals.	Labia majoria should cover the labia manoria and clitoris in the female. May have white to light pink mucousy vaginal discharge (pseudo menses).
10. Assess reflexes.	Rooting, sucking, Moro, palmar and plantar grasp. Babinski, and stepping and dancing should be present. Head lag not greater that 45 degrees.
11. Assess back and spine.	C-shaped spine, intact, no tufts of hair or fatty pads.

Key interventions and rationales

1. Place infant under a radiant warmer with skin probe attached.
   Stabilize the newborn's temperature to prevent respiratory acidosis. Prevent loss of heat through evaporation, conduction, convection, and radiation.

2. Maintain a patent airway and monitor respirations.
   The mouth and then nose should be suctioned with bulb syringe. Respirations should remain between 30 and 60 per minute. Neonates will increase their rate before respiratory depth, if compromised.

3. Provide skin integrity.
   A bath can be given when temperature is stabilized; keep cord clamped and triple tied. Clamp will remain on while cord is moist. Cord should dry, shrivel, and fall off in 7 to 10 days.

4. Administer newborn medications.
   All newborns get AquaMEPHYTON (vitamin K) 0.5 to 1 mg intramuscularly (I.M.) in the vastus lateralis on admission to nursery. All newborns get eye prophylaxis, usually erythromycin ointment. Hepatitis B immunization is offered in newborn nursery and given after parental consent.

5. Initiate preferred feeding method.
   Usually infants are given breast milk or water for the first feeding to assess for tracheal-esophageal anomalies.

6. Provide parents with follow-up care information.
   Establish follow-up visits with the health care provider. Prior to discharge, review bathing, feeding, dressing, circumcision care, and signs of illness with the parents.

High-risk newborn

<table>
<tr><td colspan="3">RISK FACTORS</td></tr>
<tr>
<td>Conditions that put the newborn at risk
• Prematurity
• Postmaturity
• Maternal diabetes mellitus
• Maternal substance abuse
• Infection
• Small-for-gestational-age (SGA) or large-for-gestational-age (LGA) status
• Hemolytic disease of the newborn
• Mechanical delivery interventions (i.e., forceps)
• Abruptio placentae</td>
<td>Problems associated with high-risk
• Neonatal morbidity
• Neonatal mortality</td>
<td>How to reduce risk
• Antepartal identification of genetic, prenatal, intrapartal, and gestational risk factors
• Labor and delivery at facility equipped to manage high-risk newborns
• Prediction of risk from Apgar scores
• Complete physical examination, gestational age assessment, and evaluation for SGA and LGA status as soon as possible after delivery</td>
</tr>
</table>

Key assessments and rationales

1. Assess risk factors.
   This determines risk level for newborn.
2. Perform physical assessment.
   This develops baseline data and alerts staff to problems requiring immediate intervention.
3. Assess the family's reaction to the newborn's condition.
   The family may experience grief and a sense of failure if they think neonate may not survive.

Key interventions with rationales

1. Monitor and support respirations.
   Immature respiratory development is the greatest problem of a preterm newborn. Monitor rate, breath sounds, cyanosis, grunting, retractions, nasal flaring, and periods of apnea. Use mechanical ventilation if necessary. Gentle handling and periodic suctioning is required with this infant. Monitor arterial blood gases for changes in oxygenation.
2. Maintain neutral thermal environment at 96.8° to 97.7° F, minimally.
   Temperature should be maintained under a radiant warmer or in an incubator. Cold stress will increase respiratory problems.
3. Monitor apical heart rate and color.
   Apical pulse may be rapid and irregular. Goal should be 120 to 160 bpm. Observe for color changes from cyanosis to pallor to

jaundice. An apnea monitor is frequently used. Parents should be taught cardiopulmonary resuscitation (CPR) prior to discharge.

4. Provide adequate nutrition.
   Small frequent feedings with increased caloric formula are given. Frequently, the newborn will need to be gavage fed because of immature suck-swallow mechanisms and easy tiring. Prevent aspiration and aspiration pneumonia.

5. Monitor hydration by measuring urinary output and weight gain.
   This assures that the neonate is receiving adequate fluids.

6. Monitor for infection.
   Premature infants have diminished passive immunity, which usually is obtained in the third trimester. They may have an increased number of invasive procedures that expose them to infection. Mandatory handwashing, aseptic technique, and minimizing exposure is necessary. Initiate prescribed antibiotic therapy as soon as an infection is identified.

7. Monitor for hypoglycemia and hypocalcemia.
   After feedings are begun, maintain venous glucose above 45 mg/dl. Jerking and tremors can mean hypocalcemia. Calcium levels need to be maintained above 7 mg/dl.

8. Monitor for risk conditions associated with preterm infants.
   Preterm infants have a greater incidence of developing shock, intraventricular hemorrhage, and circulatory failure.

9. Support the family emotionally and foster attachment behaviors.
   The family will have grief and depression as a result of birth of a preterm infant. Support them and allow touching and involving them in care as possible. Provide counseling and referral to support agencies, as needed.

Infant of a diabetic mother (IDM)

Overview

An IDM has been exposed to a high glucose level in utero and responded by increasing in size, so he will be LGA. At birth, when the high glucose levels are in decline, this infant frequently demonstrates distress to extrauterine adjustment.

Pathophysiology

In utero, the infant responded to high glucose levels by increasing insulin production. This infant will be hypoglycemic at birth. The IDM is also at high risk for respiratory distress syndrome because the increased insulin has stimulated a decrease in lecithin synthesis (L:S). LGA infants can suffer birth trauma because of their size.

Key assessments and rationales

1. Assess serum glucose levels at birth and initiate a glucose monitoring program.
   Levels should be >40 mg/dl. Initiate early feedings to maintain glucose levels, then check them at least every 4 hours for the first 24 hours.
2. Observe for signs of respiratory distress.
   Respiratory distress can result from decreased L:S ratios and prematurity.
3. Assess for birth trauma, congenital anomalies, and hypocalcemia.
   These infants are at an increased risk of birth trauma, congenital anomalies (particularly cardiac), and hypocalcemia, if premature.

Key interventions with rationales

1. Provide respiratory support as needed.
   Cold stress can lead to respiratory acidosis.
2. Initiate early feedings.
   Early feedings minimize hypoglycemia. The lethargic infant will need to be gavage fed.
3. Educate the parents about IDM.
   After initial glucose stabilization and resolving any other high-risk condition, these infants usually have no significant sequelae.

CRITICAL THINKING EXERCISE

Facts and objectives

1. The NCLEX-RN tests your ability to make sound clinical judgments.
2. Developing critical thinking skills is the foundation for being able to make good clinical judgments.
3. This exercise will help you evaluate how well you think critically.
4. As you work through this exercise, you will learn how the continuous flow of questions that evolve as you think the case through will lead you to reach solid conclusions about the client problem and the *best* nursing behaviors.

Instructions

Respond to the following questions by writing down your best thoughts, ideas and "answers" in the space provided. Do this for all of the questions, then turn the page to see what you should have considered in response to each question.

Naturally, to learn to think critically, don't look for hints or answers before completing all questions...don't cheat yourself! How you answer the critical questions will depend on how well you perfect your thinking skills.

PREGNANCY-INDUCED HYPERTENSION
Overview

A 36-year-old primigravida is 33 weeks gestation. She has come to her obstetrician for her prenatal check-up. Since her last appointment, she has gained 2 pounds, her rings are tight on her hands, and she tires easily. The obstetrician diagnoses her with pregnancy-induced hypertension (PIH), mild pre-eclampsia.

1. What are the classic triad of symptoms the nurse would associate with the diagnosis of PIH?

2. List risk factors for a client to develop PIH.

3. The client is being sent home and will be followed with home monitoring. You are to initiate her teaching plan at this time. What instructions will you give her?

The client's condition worsens after 3 days at home. She calls the office reporting a 3-pound weight gain since yesterday, blurred vision, and a continuous headache. The obstetrician orders hospital admission on the antepartal unit, with the diagnosis of PIH, severe pre-eclampsia. You are now the admission nurse on the antepartal unit for this client.

4. Utilizing a system approach, what danger signals would you look for in this client?

5. The obstetrician has ordered a loading dose of 6 g magnesium sulfate ($MgSO_4$) in 250 ml of solution I.V. over 30 minutes. As you prepare this medication, you review the classification of this drug and what will need to be monitored. What should your review consist of?

6. The client remains anxious. What is the best approach to take?

7. Three weeks later, the client begins labor. As you enter the room, you see that she is having a seizure. What actions should you take?

8. After an emergency Cesarean section, a 7-pound, 6-ounce baby boy is delivered. What effects would the $MgSO_4$ therapy have on the infant?

THE FOLLOWING ARE INTERVENTIONS AND NURSING BEHAVIORS YOU SHOULD HAVE CONSIDERED IN ANSWERING THE PREVIOUS QUESTIONS.

1. **What are the classic triad of symptoms the nurse would associate with the diagnosis of PIH?**
   - *PIH is a disease that occurs at or after 20 weeks gestation lasting until 48 hours postpartum.*
   - *Hypertension, proteinuria, and edema are the classic triad of symptoms.*
   - *The blood pressure is diagnostic if the systolic level is increased 30 mm Hg and/or the diastolic has increased 15 mm Hg. There should be two readings at a minimum of a 6-hour interval for diagnosis. If there is no baseline blood pressure available, 140/90 indicates hypertension.*
   - *Proteinuria is diagnosed as 1+ (300 mg/liter) or 2+ (1 g/liter).*
   - *Any pregnant client could have slight edema of hands and feet. It is not diagnostic. Edema of the client's face would be more significant.*

2. **List risk factors for a client to develop PIH.**
   - *Primiparous (or first pregnancy with partner), age under 16 or over 35.*
   - *Preexisting diabetes or renal disease.*
   - *Multi-gestation pregnancy.*
   - *Preexisting hypertensive disease.*

3. **The client is being sent home and will be followed with home monitoring. You are to initiate her teaching plan at this time. What instructions will you give her?**
   - *Keep a record of activities and health status, outline day-to-day activities.*
   - *Positioning--side-lying, preferably left side lying, to avoid vena cava compression and to aid in peripheral vascular circulation.*
   - *Blood pressure--monitor daily b.i.d. or t.i.d. and prn. (Parameters set by the obstetrician from the client's baseline).*
   - *Daily weight--on arising every morning (3 pounds/24 hours or 4 pounds/3 days alert).*
   - *Diet--high-protein, moderate sodium (review foods).*
   - *Fetal monitoring--kick chart and home transmission monitoring.*
   - *Urine analysis--protein dip stick q.i.d. (2+ or greater, call health care provider).*
   - *Call health care provider if not feeling well, or if headaches, blurred vision, scotomata (spots before eyes), dyspnea (difficulty breathing), or epigastric pain occur. These are all indicators that PIH is worsening and the client will need to be monitored in a more restricted environment.*

The client's condition worsens after 3 days at home. She calls the office reporting a 3-pound weight gain since yesterday, blurred vision, and a continuous headache. The obstetrician orders hospital admission on the antepartal unit, with the diagnosis of PIH, severe pre-eclampsia. You are now the admission nurse on the antepartal unit for this client.

4. **Utilizing a system approach, what danger signals would you look for in this client?**
    - *CNS--changes in state of consciousness, blurred vision, scotomata, hyperreflexia, clonus, seizure, cerebral hemorrhage.*
    - *Cardiac system--hypertension, increased cardiac workload, cardiac decompensation.*
    - *Hematologic system--decreased platelet count ($<100,000 \ mm^3$).*
    - *Hepatic system--nausea, vomiting, epigastric pain.*
    - *Respiratory system--decreased respirations, dyspnea, pulmonary edema.*
    - *Renal system--decreased renal perfusion and glomerular filtration (decreased urinary output), increased serum creatine level and uric acid level, proteinuria, and late hematuria.*

5. **The obstetrician has ordered a loading dose of 6 g magnesium sulfate ($MgSO_4$) in 250 ml of solution I.V. over 30 minutes. As you prepare this medication, you review the classification of this drug and what will need to be monitored. What should your review consist of?**
    - *$MgSO_4$ is classified as a CNS depressant. It is given to PIH clients to reduce the risk of convulsion. The blood pressure is reduced as a secondary response because of relaxation of smooth muscles.*
    - *$MgSO_4$ is contraindicated in a client with myasthenia gravis. Clients with cardiac and/or renal impairment need to be watched very closely.*
    - *There needs to be close, consistent monitoring of the client's sensorium, blood pressure, serum magnesium levels (4 to 8 mg/dl), respiratory rate (>12/minute), patellar reflex ($1+$ or greater), clonus, urinary output (>30 ml/hr), FHT (120 to 160 bpm)*
    - *Calcium gluconate (1 g I.V. over 3 minutes) is the drug antagonist for magnesium sulfate and should readily be available.*

6. **The client remains anxious. What is the best approach to take?**
    - *Calm and reassure the client that she is in the best environment for her and the baby.*
    - *The only "cure" for PIH is delivery. Monitor the client for 48 hours after delivery.*

7. **Three weeks later the client begins labor. As you enter the room, you see the client having a seizure. What actions should you take?**
    - *Position her in a safe area turned on her side to maintain a patent airway.*
    - *Call for assistance.*
    - *Administer oxygen, as necessary.*
    - *Assess and document time of onset and length of seizure, parts of body involved, maternal vital signs, fetal activity and FHT, incontinence, and indications of abruptio placentae.*

8. **After an emergency Cesarean section, a 7-pound, 6-ounce baby boy is delivered. What effects would the $MgSO_4$ therapy have on the infant?**
    - *$MgSO_4$ readily crosses the placental barrier but does not present risk factors to the fetus.*
    - *The problems of respiratory and neurological depression this infant may experience is due to perinatal asphyxia as a result of the mother's seizure and Cesarean delivery.*

CHAPTER *6*

VIEW THE PROGRAM *"GROWTH & DEVELOPMENT"* BEFORE PROCEEDING. IT IS THE 5TH PROGRAM ON THE VIDEO MODULE.

TRACHEOESOPHAGEAL FISTULA/ESOPHAGEAL ATRESIA

Overview

Tracheoesophageal fistula (TEF) and esophageal atresia (EA) are congenital malformations caused by a failure of the trachea and esophagus to separate into distinct structures (TEF) and a failure of the esophagus to develop as a continuous channel (EA) during the fourth and fifth week of gestation. These defects may occur as individual entities or in combination, and without early diagnosis and prompt treatment they pose a threat to the infant's life. The incidence of the defects is approximately 1 in 3,500 births. A large percentage of affected infants are premature or of low birth weight. There is a history of maternal polyhydramnios. More than 40% of the infants have other anomalies, including congenital heart disease, anorectal malformations, pulmonary and renal anomalies, and vertebral and limb defects.

Pathophysiology

During the 4th to 5th of gestation, the foregut normally lengthens and separates, forming two parallel tubes (the esophagus and trachea) connected only at the larynx. Any interruption in this process leads to esophageal or tracheal anomalies.

The esophageal defect may consist of two blind pouches, one at the pharyngeal end and one at the gastric end, or one portion ends in a blind pouch and the other portion is connected to the trachea via a fistula. The most common type consists of a blind pouch of the upper esophageal segment and a fistula between the lower esophageal segment and the trachea. The gap between the upper and lower segments generally is small and primary surgical correction usually is successful. The second most common type is characterized by a blind pouch at each end of the esophagus, widely separated and with no communication to the trachea. Other forms of the defects may be an intact esophagus with a TEF or an EA, with fistulas between the upper or lower esophageal segments and the trachea.

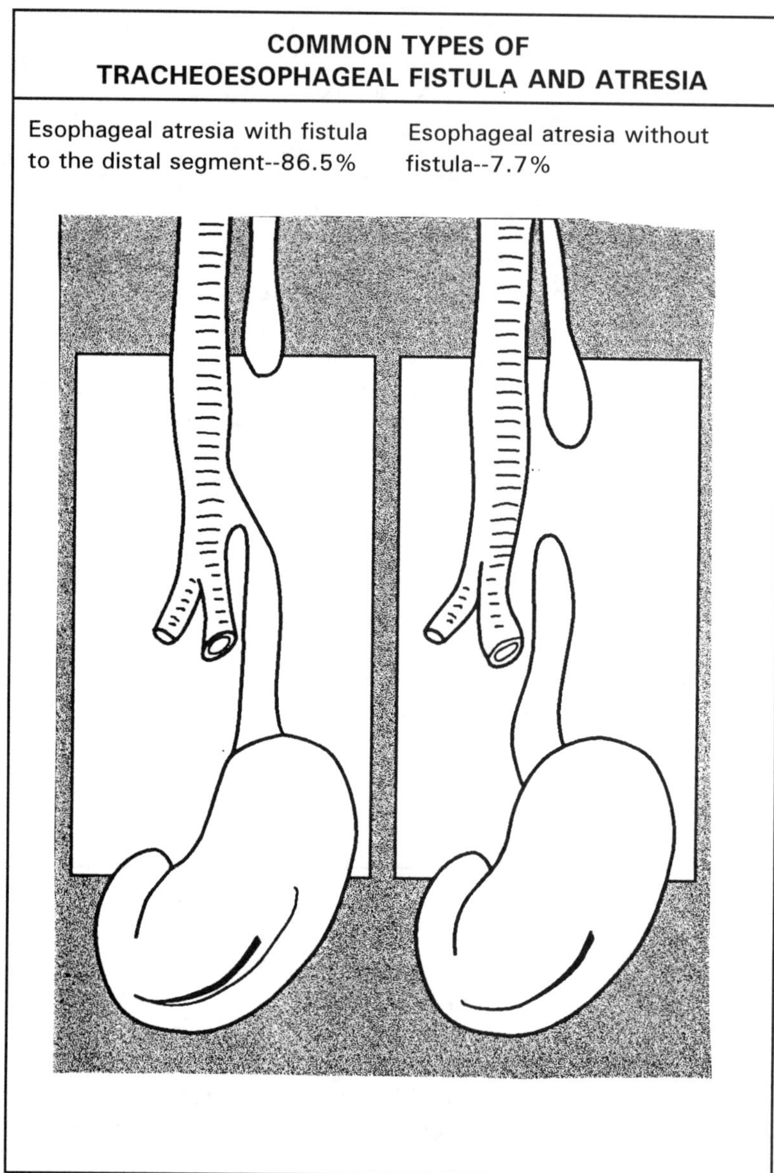

Key assessments and rationales

1. Perform a complete newborn assessment.
   Assess the infant's general state of health and identify any congenital anomalies.

2. Observe the infant for excessive frothy salivation in the mouth and nose, drooling, coughing, choking, cyanosis, and apnea.
   These are the classic clinical manifestations of TEF and EA.
3. Assess the infant's respiratory status frequently.
   Infants with TEF and EA are at high risk for respiratory distress.

Key interventions and rationales
Preoperative
1. Keep infant under a radiant warmer, and administer humidified, warmed oxygen.
   This maintains a neutral thermal environment and helps relieve respiratory distress.
2. Keep the infant NPO.
   This will prevent aspiration.
3. Suction the infant as necessary.
   This removes accumulated secretions from oropharynx.
4. Maintain low, intermittent suction of esophageal segment of the defect with a double-lumen catheter.
   This will keep the blind pouch empty.
5. Position the infant supine with his head elevated at least 30 degrees on an inclined plane.
   This decreases pressure on thoracic cavity and minimizes reflux of gastric secretions up the distal esophagus and into the trachea and bronchi.
6. Initiate I.V. fluids, monitor I&O, urine specific gravity, and weight.
   Maintain hydration and monitor fluid balance.
7. Institute broad-spectrum antibiotic therapy.
   Aspiration pneumonia is almost inevitable and appears early.

Postoperative
1. Monitor the infant's respiratory status.
   Identify early manifestations of distress.
2. Monitor the infant's weight, I&O, skin turgor, mucus membranes, and anterior fontanel.
   These are the best indicators of hydration status.
3. Maintain fluid balance and nutrition.
   This prevents dehydration.
4. Maintain a neutral thermal environment, using a radiant warmer or an isolette with "servo" control.
   Cold can negatively affect a newborn's respiratory status.

5. Provide meticulous skin care at ostomy site.
   This prevents skin breakdown and infection.
6. Encourage parents to participate in the infant's care.
   This provides comfort and security and promotes parent-infant bonding.
7. Suction the infant using a catheter pre-measured so it does not reach the surgical site.
   This will prevent trauma to suture line.
8. Teach the family the skills they will need for home care: positioning, suctioning, dressing changes, gastrostomy feedings, care of ostomy site, and signs of complications and respiratory distress.
   This ensures continuity of care after discharge. Parents need to be prepared for home care to avoid unnecessary anxiety in caring for their infant.

Drugs commonly used in this disorder
1. Prophylactic broad-spectrum antibiotics, preoperatively and postoperatively, as the infant is at risk for aspiration pneumonia.

Nutrition considerations
1. Preoperatively, maintain I.V. fluids.
2. Postoperatively, keep the infant on parenteral nutrition until he can tolerate oral feedings, usually on the 5th to 7th postop day.
3. Prior to gastrostomy feedings, the tube is elevated and secured at a point above the level of the stomach, allowing gastric secretions to the duodenum, while swallowed air can escape through open tube, preventing irritation to the suture line.
4. After gastrostomy feedings, keep the tube elevated and unclamped to allow for passage of air or regurgitation.
5. When esophageal anastomosis is healed, begin PO feedings with sterile water, followed by small frequent feedings of formula or breast milk.

MYELOMENINGOCELE

Overview

Myelomeningocele is a hernial protrusion of a saclike cyst of meninges, spinal fluid, and a portion of the spinal cord with its nerves through a bony defect in the vertebral column because the neural plate fails to close as it forms the neural tube during the first 28 days of pregnancy. Prenatal detection is possible between weeks 14 to 22 using alpha-fetoprotein levels, but positive confirmation requires amniocentesis and ultrasonography. It can also be detected at birth and accounts for 90% of spinal cord lesions. Myelomeningocele may be located at any point along the spinal column. A fine membrane that can tear easily and leak cerebrospinal fluid, it usually covers the sac or it may be encased by dura, meninges, or skin. The etiology in most cases is unknown, although there is evidence to suggest a genetic predisposition. Folic acid deficiency in the mother has been linked to neural tube defects.

Pathophysiology
Neural tube formation begins in the cervical region and progresses in both directions until, by the end of the 4th gestational week, the boundaries of the neural tube are closed. Spina bifida occulta must be present before myelomeningocele lesions can occur. The degree of impairment is related to the size and level of the defect on the spinal cord. Among spinal cord lesions, 90% are at L-2 and below. The lesion results in flaccid paralysis or partial paralysis of the lower extremities and varying degrees of motor, sensory, reflex, and sphincter dysfunction. Talipes valgus or varus contractures, kyphosis, lumbosacral scoliosis, and hip dislocations may be associated with the defect. Associated malformations may include hydrocephalus and Arnold-Chiari malformation.

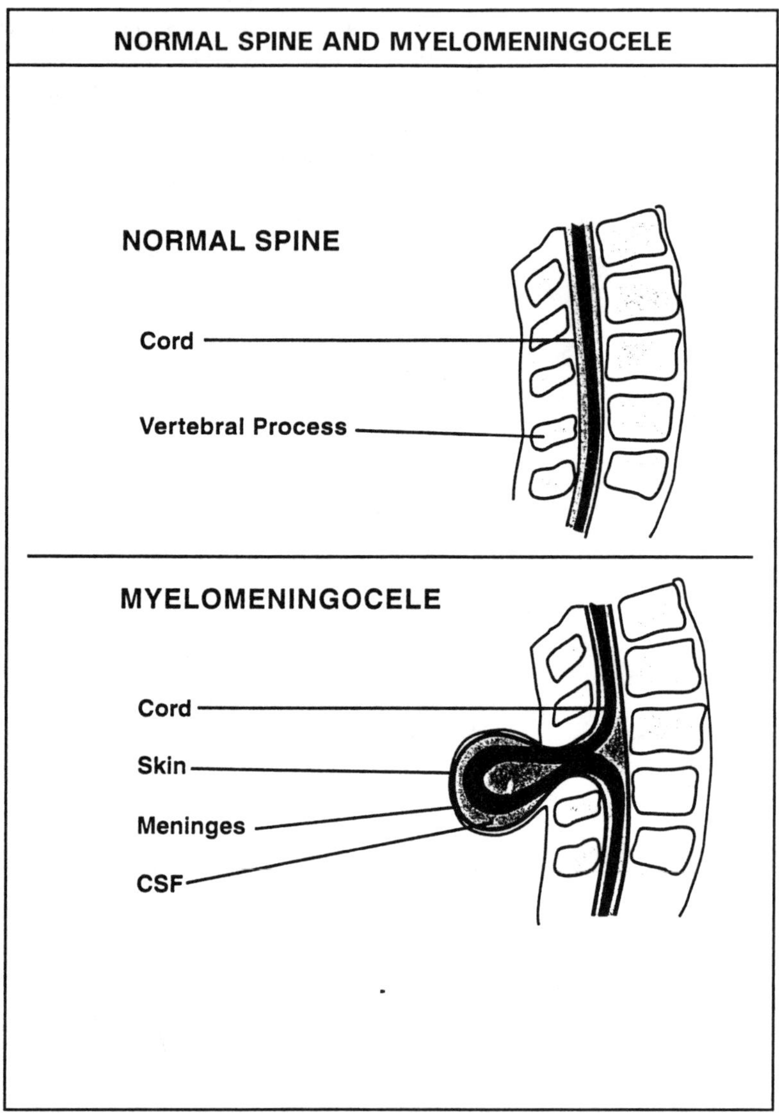

Key assessments and rationales

1. Perform a physical assessment.
   Assess the infant's general state of health and identify if any associated joint deformities are present.

2. Assess for a visible sac, sensory disturbances and deficits, overflow incontinence with constant dribbling of urine, poor anal sphincter tone, and poor anal skin tone.

These are the clinical manifestations of myelomeningocele.
3. Perform a neurological assessment.
   Determine the level of motor and sensory impairment.
4. Assess for abnormal head circumference or rapid head growth, tense or bulging anterior fontanel, separation of cranial sutures, dilated scalp veins, thinning of skull bones, irritability, lethargy, difficulty in feeding, vomiting, high-pitched cry, increased blood pressure, and decreased apical rate.
   These are the signs and symptoms of hydrocephalus and increasing intracranial pressure.
5. Inspect myelomeningocele sac for abrasions, tears, redness, and purulent drainage.
   Redness and drainage may indicate infection. Abrasions and tears could lead to infection.
6. Monitor vital signs and general behavior.
   An elevated or subnormal temperature, irritability, pallor, and vomiting may be early signs of a meningeal infection.

Key interventions and rationales
1. Assess the infant's skin, gently massaging it during bathing and handle carefully.
   This is to assess for irritation, to increase circulation, and to prevent damage to sac or surgical site.
2. Change diaper pads as soon as soiled, and clean genital area frequently, applying protective devices around sac.
   This keeps the skin clean, dry, free of irritation, and prevents contamination of sac from waste.
3. Position the infant prone on pressure-reducing mattress with her head turned to side.
   This helps protect the sac and prevents pressure ulcers.
4. Maintain hip abduction with pad or sandbag.
   This will prevent hip dislocation.
5. Keep the infant's feet in a neutral position with a small roll under the ankles.
   This will prevent contractures.
6. Apply sterile, saline-soaked dressings (at body temperature) over the sac preoperatively.
   This will prevent drying of sac.
7. Monitor urinary output for retention and ensure adequate fluid intake.
   This will minimize risk of infection caused by stasis of urine, increase urination, and prevent bacterial growth.

8. Assess fontanels and measure occipitofrontal circumference every shift.
   This will detect increased intracranial pressure and developing hydrocephalus.
9. Talk to the infant while providing care. Play music and recordings of family voices, and place brightly colored objects within visual field.
   Provide visual and auditory stimulation to maintain the infant's developmental level.
10. Encourage the family to caress, speak, and participate in the infant's care.
    This will promote bonding.
11. Teach the family skills they will need for home care, such as skin care, range-of-motion exercises, intermittent clean catheterization, bowel and bladder programs, and signs of hydrocephalus, and provide a diet adequate in fluid and fiber.
    To ensure appropriate care after discharge, parents need to be prepared for caring for their infant at home.
12. Refer the parents to community health nurses and support groups, such as the Spina Bifida Association of America.
    The care of the child with myelomeningocele can be overwhelming because of primary concerns and associated problems. These organizations can provide resources, educational materials, and emotional support to families.

Drugs commonly used in this disorder
1. Prophylactic antibiotics may be used preoperatively and postoperatively and to vigorously treat meningitis, UTI, and pneumonia.

Nutrition considerations
1. Feed in side-lying position, preoperatively, being careful not to injure sac. Burp by gently rubbing between shoulder blades, above the sac.
2. Postoperatively, hold the infant for feedings, with careful burping and bubbling performed in the preop manner until the suture line has healed.

ASTHMA

Overview

Asthma or reactive airway disease (RAD) is a chronic pulmonary condition and the most frequent admitting diagnosis in children's hospitals. Asthma's frequency, severity, and mortality appears to be on the rise, with the onset of childhood asthma occurring by age 2 in more than 50% of cases and by age 5 in 80% of afflicted children. Asthma is airway obstruction characterized by bronchial irritability after exposure to various stimuli. It may reverse spontaneously or with treatment.

An exacerbation of asthma may be precipitated after exposure to a variety of stimuli, such as specific allergens, irritants (including secondhand smoke), respiratory infections, exercise, weather changes, or from emotional upset. The immature anatomy of infants and small children predisposes them to increased distress from asthma. Their smaller, narrower airway and decreased elastic lung recoil makes them more prone to airway obstruction. The child's flexible rib cage and underdeveloped chest muscle and diaphragm lead to exhaustion with increased respiratory effort. The severity of asthma often decreases with age because of increased airway size, improved diaphragm support, and more efficient mucus clearing.

Pathophysiology

Asthma is characterized by bronchospasm, inflammation, and edema of the mucus membranes, accumulation of viscous secretions, and increased airway responsiveness to diverse stimuli. The resulting airway narrowing may be partial or complete, leading to impaired ventilation and gas exchange. If these physiologic responses are not reversed early, air becomes trapped in the alveoli, causing air hunger and resultant hyperinflation. The blocked inspired air and poor gas exchange progressively leads to hypoxia and acidosis. During the early stage, the hypoxemia and metabolic acidosis may be compensated by the child's increased respiratory rate. As the episode progresses, a combined respiratory and metabolic acidosis develops. The respiratory acidosis is caused by increased carbon dioxide retention, and the metabolic acidosis is a result of anaerobic metabolism, ketosis, and an accumulation of metabolites.

Key assessments and rationales

1. Obtain a family health history and a thorough current health history, including onset of symptoms, history of cough, upper

respiratory infection, bronchospasm or wheezing, and exposure to known allergens.

Among children with severe asthma, 40% have one parent similarly affected. A thorough health history is necessary, including the use and effect of asthma medications previously used. Prior hospitalizations should be documented because past experiences may affect the child's perception of the present illness.

2. Assess the child for cough, presence of wheezing, shortness of breath, dyspnea on exertion, prolonged expirations, restlessness, anxiety, diaphoresis, and evidence of cyanosis.
   These are the signs and symptoms of an asthma episode, with restlessness, anxiety, and cyanosis being signs of hypoxia.

3. Obtain baseline vital signs and auscultate breath sounds, noting any adventitious sounds, areas of diminished air entry, assess respiratory rate and effort, presence of retractions, use of accessory muscles, nasal flaring, pulse oximetry values, and observe color frequently.
   Subtle changes in the child's condition may serve as an early warning of increased airway obstruction.

4. Assess the child's level of consciousness and general behavior.
   These are important indicators of oxygenation. As infants and children become more hypoxic, they may not interact appropriately with their parents, who immediately note the behavioral change. Failure to resist or cry during painful procedures is an ominous sign.

5. Assess the child's hydration status: fluid intake, urine output and urine specific gravity, body weight, mucous membranes, skin turgor, and presence of tears.
   Tachypnea, diaphoresis, and decreased intake of oral fluids may cause dehydration.

6. Assess the family's knowledge of the disease and its management and the degree of their cooperation.
   This provides the basis for future teaching.

Key interventions and rationales

1. Monitor the child's vital signs every 15 to 30 minutes, observing for signs of hypoxia.
   Subtle changes in the child's condition may be an early warning of increased airway obstruction.

2. Administer humidified oxygen; if child has chronic carbon dioxide retention do not exceed 2 liters/minute.
   Supplemental oxygen decreases hypoxia that occurs from airway edema, mucus, and bronchospasm; administering oxygen to a child with chronic carbon dioxide retention may lead to

respiratory depression by decreasing stimulus to breathe.
3. Keep the child in an upright position.
   An upright position aids in lung expansion and decreases pressure on the diaphragm.
4. Maintain an I.V. infusion, correcting dehydration slowly.
   Fluid therapy helps liquefy secretions and replaces fluids lost through tachypnea. Overhydration can obstruct small airways from accumulation of interstitial fluid.
5. Maintain NPO status.
   This will decrease the risk of aspiration.
6. Provide humidified environment.
   Humidification helps liquefy secretions and promotes hydration.
7. Keep parents and child informed of condition in an age-appropriate manner.
   Knowledge decreases anxiety and gives parents and child a sense of control.
8. Encourage the child to deep breathe and cough.
   Respiratory treatments and exercises help free and expel secretions and re-expand lung tissue. Mucus plugs can lead to atelectasis.
9. Maintain a peaceful, quiet environment. Encourage the parents' presence.
   Anxiety increases bronchospasm. Parents' presence decreases the child's fear and anxiety.
10. Teach the child and parents about drug regime, use of inhalers, and the difference between maintenance and acute exacerbation therapy. Teach the child age-appropriate management skills.
    This will ensure appropriate care post discharge.
11. Teach the child and parents the importance of a healthy lifestyle.
    Regular exercise, adequate fluids and nutrition, rest, and preventing infection promote pulmonary and cardiovascular health and help the child lead a normal life.

Drugs commonly used in this disorder
1. Albuterol (Proventil)--this bronchodilator relaxes bronchial smooth muscle and inhibits the release of mediators from mast cells. Dose range: Based on body weight: usually 0.3 to 6.0 mg/kg/24 hours in divided doses, t.i.d. Nursing considerations include baseline vital signs and monitoring frequently during therapy; maintaining the child on cardiopulmonary monitor; explaining use of inhaler; offering sips of water for dry mouth.
2. Cromolyn sodium (Intal)--this inhaled nonsteroidal, anti-inflammatory drug prevents asthma symptoms by blocking the

release of mast cell mediators. Dose range: Children over 2 years, two inhales from an aerosol inhaler, q.i.d.; children over 5 years, 20-mg capsules q6h via Spinhaler. Nursing considerations include teaching the child to use the drug only as prescribed because it will not help during an acute asthma episode and may worsen symptoms; offering sips of water before and gum and oral hygiene after inhalation to reduce cough, irritation, bad taste, and dryness; and teaching use and care of inhaler. The capsules are contracted for children with lactose intolerance.

Nutrition considerations

1. Small frequent feedings at room temperature, as tolerated to avoid abdominal distention, which might interfere with diaphragmatic excursion.
2. Avoid milk and milk products during asthma episode because they can increase coughing and mucus production.
3. Upon discharge, tell the child to drink three to eight glasses (750 to 2,000 ml) of fluid a day to decrease the viscosity of secretions.

CLEFT LIP AND CLEFT PALATE

Overview

Cleft lip (CL) and cleft palate (CP) are congenital anomalies that are evident at birth. They may occur unilaterally or bilaterally, but both result from embryologic failures in development because of multiple genetic and environmental factors. The result is an abnormal opening in the lip, palate, and in some cases, nose. Each of these abnormalities appear as distinct malformations, but they also may appear together.

Pathophysiology

Cleft lip is a cleft, or open space, between the nasal cavity and lip. The extent of the cleft varies greatly from an indentation in the lip to a deep, wide fissure extending to the nostril. With bilateral CL, the mid-portion of the upper lip is unattached on either side and may be displaced forward. It may or may not be associated with CP, which varies greatly in degree; it may involve only the soft palate or extend into the hard palate and other structures forming the palate (uvula, maxillary teeth). The cleft may occur only in the midline of the posterior palate or extend to the nostrils. Wide, central clefts may be accompanied by partial or complete absence of nasal septal development, resulting in open communication between the nasal and oral cavities.

Key assessments and rationales

1. Perform a physical assessment.
   Assess the newborn's general health and identify any other congenital anomalies.
2. Inspect the infant's palate, visually and by placing gloved hand or finger directly on palate.
   Assess the degree of the defect.
3. Assess degree of cleft and any sucking impairment.
   Infants with cleft lip alone or simple cleft dental arch may succeed at breast or bottle feeding, without interventions.
4. Observe the infant's feeding behavior and his parents' ability and comfort level in feeding him.
   Determine the infant's ability to suck and swallow. Parents' knowledge and ability to feed infant will determine what kind of teaching plan will be needed.
5. Observe interactions between the infant and his parents.
   This will assess the degree of parents' acceptance of the infant and give information about the kind of support the parents may need.

Key interventions and rationales

1. Let the parents express their feelings. Convey an attitude of acceptance of infant and family; encourage touching and holding.
   Expressing feelings about their infant's anomaly will help the parents develop coping skills. Parents are sensitive to the attitudes of others. Touching encourages bonding and prevents a delayed attachment.
2. Explain corrective surgical procedure to the parents, using photographs of satisfactory results.
   This will encourage positive feelings of the eventual outcome.
3. Postoperatively, position the infant on his back or in an infant seat designed for CL repair.
   This will prevent trauma to operative site.
4. Maintain a protective lip device.
   Protective devices like the Logan bar prevent separation of the lip suture lines.
5. Use elbow restraints postoperatively for both CL and CP repair. Remove restraints periodically while parents or nurse stay with the infant.
   Restraints prevent accessing the operative site. They need to be removed to exercise arms, to do range of motion, and to assess skin integrity and circulation.
6. Clean suture line gently with sterile water or saline, using a cotton

swab and a rolling motion from the suture line out, after feeding. Teach parents cleansing technique.
This decreases risk for infection; it removes crusting and minimizes scarring.

7. Avoid placing anything in the infant's mouth after a CP repair. Do not brush the child's teeth for 1 or 2 weeks postop; rinse mouth with water after feedings to clean palate repair.
This will prevent trauma to operative site and accidental tear of palatal sutures. Rinsing food and residual sugars from suture line reduces the risk of infection.

8. Provide pain-relief and comfort measures. Have parents cuddle, hold, rock, and talk to the infant.
This relieves discomfort, increases parental involvement, and promotes optimum growth and development.

9. Monitor for signs of infection.
Infection must be identified early because inflammation can increase scarring.

10. Encourage the parents to share concerns about long-term care and refer them to support groups.
Cleft disorders are long-term health problems that require extensive follow-up, straining the family's resources. By identifying concerns early, care options can be discussed. Support groups can provide useful resources to aid in care.

Drugs commonly used in this disorder
1. There are no specific drugs used in these disorders.

Nutrition considerations
1. Assist the mother with breast-feeding--many infants with either defect can still breast-feed.
2. Provide alternative assistive feeding devices (lamb's nipple, gravity flow nipple, flanged nipple Breck feeder, Asepto syringe) as needed, to compensate for infant's feeding difficulty.
3. Feed the infant in an upright position and burp and bubble him frequently, because infants with CL and CP have a tendency to swallow excessive amounts of air.
4. Monitor the infant's weight to assess adequacy of nutritional intake.
5. Provide emotional support to parents as they learn to feed their child, as self-care and bonding are improved when parents can assume total care.

DEVELOPMENTAL DYSPLASIA OF THE HIP

Overview

Developmental dysplasia of the hip (DDH), formally called congenital hip dysplasia (CHD) or congenital dislocation of the hip, describes a group of disorders related to abnormal development of the hip in which there is a shallow acetabulum, subluxation, or dislocation. There is wide range of severity of hip dysplasia, ranging from very mild to severely dislocated. It may be congenital, but in some children it develops after birth, consequently the term developmental dysplasia of the hip. One fifth of the cases seen involve both hips. When it is unilateral, the left hip is affected three times more often than the right hip. If the condition is diagnosed early, the femoral head usually can be returned to the normal position easily. After reducing the femoral head, it must be maintained within the acetabulum until the joint capsule returns to its normal configuration.

Pathophysiology

The etiology of DDH is unknown, although some predisposing factors have been identified. There is a family history of the defect in about 33% of the cases. The disorder occurs more often in females and firstborn children and is more prevalent in infants carried or delivered in breech position. Maternal estrogens and hormones affecting maternal pelvic laxity prior to birth may temporarily cause laxity of the pelvic joint and hip capsule in a newborn and lead to joint instability.

At birth, the ball and joint sockets of the hip are chiefly cartilaginous. As ossification of the hip proceeds, the head of the femur must be contained within the acetabulum for normal hip configuration to develop. If the head of the femur is not positioned well within the joint, adaptive changes cause varying degrees of deformity in the femur, acetabulum, soft tissues, and joint capsule.

Key assessments and rationales

1. Perform a newborn assessment.
   Assess his general health state and determine if other musculoskeletal defects are present.
2. Assess the infant for apparent shortening of femur on affected side, asymmetry of gluteal or thigh folds, with deeper creases on affected side, limited abduction of the affected hip.
   These are the classic clinical manifestations of developmental hip dysplasia.

3. Perform Ortolani maneuver. (This should be done only by experienced RN or health care provider.)
   Assess for dislocation of the hip upon abduction in infant under 4 weeks old.

Key interventions and rationales

1. Demonstrate and teach the parents the proper care, use, and/or application of a Pavlik harness or spica cast, including feeding and bathing techniques.
   Corrective devices hold the femoral head in the acetabulum.
   Improper application of the device could cause avascular necrosis; incorrect use of the harness straps can cause skin irritation.
   Parents need to be confident and comfortable with these skills.
2. Teach the parents how to hold, nurse, and cuddle the infant while confined to the harness or cast.
   This will promote parent/infant bonding.
3. Teach the parents how to protect the infant's skin and legs under the harness.
   Using protective layers of clothing, such as undershirts and long socks will reduce skin irritation.
4. Perform bilateral neurovascular checks while the infant is in the corrective device.
   Neurovascular checks include assessing motion, color, pain, temperature, capillary refill, pedal pulses, edema, sensation, tingling, and numbness. Snug corrective devices can cause tissue swelling and circulatory compromise in the affected extremity.
5. Teach the parents how to place disposable diapers under the edges of the perineal opening in a spica cast.
   Excess urine can trickle under the cast, irritating and macerating the skin and becoming malodorous.
6. Emphasize the importance of meticulous hygiene and skin care; massage the skin at least once a day.
   Damp or moist skin inside a cast is an excellent environment for bacterial growth. Skin that is clean and dry is less likely to break down. Frequent massage increases circulation.
7. Teach parents to report fever, wound drainage, signs of discomfort, coolness or paleness of the feet, decreased motion of the legs or feet, and swelling.
   Parents must be alert to the early signs of infection and neurovascular impairment.
8. Give the parents information about car seat restraints that are available for the child in a Pavlik harness or spica cast.
   This ensures the child's safety while traveling in a car.

Drugs commonly used in this disorder
1. There are no specific drugs used in this disorder.

Nutrition considerations
1. A diet high in calories, calcium, and protein with increased dietary fiber and fluid intake will prevent constipation while the child is in spica cast and promote healing and bone development.

BRONCHIOLITIS

Overview

Bronchiolitis is an inflammation of the bronchioles. It is a lower respiratory tract illness resulting from an infecting agent that causes inflammation and obstruction of the bronchioles. It is commonly caused by the respiratory syncytial virus (RSV), but may also be caused by the parainfluenza virus, enterovirus, influenza virus, rhinovirus, adenovirus, or by a bacterial organism. Infection from more than one of the viruses may occur simultaneously.

Bronchiolitis occurs most often in winter and early spring in children under age 2, with the highest incidence seen within the first 2 to 12 months of age. Some infants and children have mild symptoms and are easily managed at home; others become acutely ill with severe respiratory distress that can become a life-threatening emergency. Infection tends to be most severe in infants under 6 months of age, and they are routinely hospitalized when bronchiolitis is diagnosed.

Pathophysiology

Viral inflammation of the bronchioles results in edema of the airway passages and eventual accumulation of mucus and exudate from cellular destruction. The bronchioles become occluded, some partially and others totally. The alveoli usually are normal, except those in the immediate vicinity of the inflamed bronchioles. The edema and exudate further compromise bronchial passages that normally narrow during expiration, trapping air in the alveoli. Infants with bronchiolitis can take in enough air but may have trouble expelling it, resulting in hyperinflation of the lungs and air trapping. This creates the wheezing and crackles heard upon auscultation and the hyperinflated or barrel chest that is a classic sign of bronchiolitis. Air trapped below the obstruction interferes with normal gas exchange. The impaired ventilation can result in hypoxemia and hypercapnia, leading to respiratory acidosis.

Key assessments and rationales

1. Obtain a complete health history.
   Children with bronchiolitis usually have a 1- to 3-day history of upper respiratory infection and low-grade fever. Risk factors include prematurity, low birth weight, congenital anomalies, and congenital heart disease.
2. Assess the home environment.
   A family history of asthma, maternal smoking and smoking in the home, overcrowding, and low socioeconomic status contribute to the risks.
3. Assess for tachypnea, dyspnea, retractions, nasal flaring, and cyanosis.
   These are common signs and symptoms of respiratory distress.
4. Assess heart rate, rhythm, blood pressure, pulses, and perfusion.
   Acutely ill infants who are tachypneic and feeding poorly are at risk for hypovolemia.
5. Check mucous membranes, urine output, urine specific gravity, anterior fontanel, and weight.
   These will provide data on hydration status.
6. Assess level of consciousness.
   This is an important indicator of whether adequate oxygenation is being received.

Key interventions and rationales

1. Monitor respirations and auscultate breath sounds.
   This determines quality of aeration and provides information about possible changes, such as increasing obstruction.
2. Monitor vital signs q2-4h and prn.
   Hypoxia causes an increase in pulse, respirations, and blood pressure.
3. Administer humidified oxygen, as ordered.
   Oxygen decreases hypoxia. Humidification liquefies mucus and decreases bronchial edema.
4. Position head at 30 to 40 degrees with neck slightly extended.
   This maintains an open airway and eases breathing by decreasing pressure on diaphragm.
5. Use cardiopulmonary monitor and pulse oximeter.
   Cardiopulmonary monitors alarm if child has a period of apnea longer than 15 or 20 seconds. Pulse oximetry continuously monitors oxygen saturation.
6. Perform chest physiotherapy.

Regular use of chest physiotherapy loosens mucus obstructing the airways, easing its removal.
7. Schedule care to allow for rest periods.
Oxygen needs decrease during rest periods.
8. Monitor I.V. fluids and, if no signs of respiratory distress, encourage oral fluids.
This helps liquefy secretions and prevents dehydration.
9. Monitor I&O and weigh the child daily.
I&O measurement helps assess hydration and fluid replacement needs. Short-term weight changes are the most reliable indicator of fluid loss or gain.

Drugs commonly used with this disorder
1. Ribavirin (Virazole)--this antiviral respiratory drug interferes with RNA and DNA synthesis, inhibiting viral replication. Dose range: 20 mg/ml, delivered via Viratek Small Particle Aerosol Generator, resulting in mist concentration of 190 mg/liters at a flow rate of 12.5 liters of mist per minute over 12 to 18 hours for 3 to 7 days. Nursing considerations include obtaining baseline vital signs and monitoring frequently; warning women who are pregnant, lactating, or pursuing conception within 6 weeks to avoid contact with the drug; putting children in a private room with the door closed and post signs alerting staff and visitors; wearing respirator mask, gown, gloves, hair and shoe covers when in the room; washing hands before leaving the room; wearing goggles--and making sure that visitors wearing contact lenses wear goggles.

Nutrition considerations
1. During periods of tachypnea, nutrition should be by I.V. therapy or nasogastric tube feedings.
2. When the child is not in respiratory distress, small, frequent oral feedings may be given.

DIARRHEA

Overview
Diarrhea is one of the most common disorders in childhood, affecting more than 50 million children worldwide every year. It is defined as an increase in the frequency, fluidity, and volume of stools. It may be acute or chronic, inflammatory or noninflammatory.

Acute diarrhea is usually self-limiting, lasting from a few days to a week. Diarrhea that lasts longer than 3 weeks most likely is related to malabsorption. Viral gastroenteritis is the most common cause of diarrhea in children over 1 year old. If untreated, it can lead to dehydration, acid-base imbalances, electrolyte imbalance, and hypovolemic shock. Acute diarrhea can be life-threatening in infants and small children if fluid loss is not replaced.

Pathophysiology
Increased motility and rapid emptying of the intestines results in impaired absorption of nutrients and water and electrolytes. Water, sodium, potassium, and bicarbonate are drawn from the extracellular space into the stool, resulting in dehydration, electrolyte depletion, and metabolic acidosis. Diarrhea occurs when there is excess fluid in the small intestine caused by bacteria that stimulate the transport of electrolytes into the small intestine, causing the cells of the mucosal lining to become irritated and secrete water and electrolytes. In other situations, bacterial or viral organisms invade and destroy intestinal mucosal cells, decreasing the surface area and impairing the intestine's ability to absorb fluids and electrolytes.

Key assessments and rationales
1. Assess the child for fever, abdominal cramping, headache, nausea, and vomiting.
   These symptoms often accompany diarrhea.
2. Obtain health information about family members, household pets, or contact with animals.
   Diarrhea can be transmitted from family members, pets, and animals such as turtles, reptiles, hamsters, dogs, and cats.
3. Assess the child's diet and any dietary changes.
   Food intolerance, allergy, hyperosmolar formulas, "sorbitol" in sugar-free gum, dietary indiscretions, or contamination can cause diarrhea.
4. Obtain information about recent travel, especially outside the United States.
   Diarrhea can be transmitted from ingesting contaminated water.
5. Assess stool patterns, including a description of the number of stools, consistency, odor, and presence of mucus or blood.
   Diarrhea stools usually are of sudden onset, profuse, watery, bloody with mucus, and foul smelling.
6. Assess state of dehydration.
   Fewer wet diapers than normal, no tears when crying, irritability,

high-pitched cry, difficult to awaken, increased respiratory rate or difficulty in breathing, depressed fontanel, sunken eyes with dark circles, abnormal color, skin turgor, temperature, or dryness are the signs and symptoms of dehydration in infants and children.

Key interventions and rationales
1. Weigh the child on the same scale and at the same time each day.
   Weight is a valuable indicator of hydration status.
2. Monitor and document I&O hourly; weigh diapers after each soiling; and monitor urine color and specific gravity q2-4h.
   I&O and specific gravity are indicators of hydration status. Urine output should be at least 2 ml/kg for infants and toddlers and 1 ml/kg for school-age children. Each gram increase of diaper weight is equivalent to 1 ml of urine.
3. Monitor the child's vital signs q2-4h. Do not take temperature rectally.
   Dehydration can quickly lead to shock in infants and small children. A rectal thermometer can stimulate peristalsis and cause more diarrhea.
4. Observe and document the amount, frequency, color, and consistency of stools.
   This helps determine the need for fluid and electrolyte replacement and helps note any changes or improvement in the child's condition.
5. Administer fluids, as prescribed.
   Excessive output without replacement leads to fluid deficit and electrolyte imbalance.
6. Assess hydration status q2-4h.
   Dehydration can develop rapidly in infants and small children.
7. Implement body substance isolation and teach visitors and family protective measures, especially handwashing.
   This will prevent the spread of infection.
8. Monitor for skin breakdown.
   Skin breakdown increases the risk for infection.
9. Teach family good hand-washing technique, diaper changing, using the toilet, and proper food preparation.
   These precautions will help prevent future episodes of diarrhea.

Drugs commonly used with this disorder
1. Antibiotics if caused by bacterial agent.

Nutrition considerations

1. Frequent clear liquids, in small amounts, at room temperature for older children and oral rehydration solutions, such as Pedialyte or Infalyte for infants and younger children.
2. Omit or limit apple juice because the high osmolality can cause loose stools.
3. Avoid sugary drinks because they lack the necessary electrolytes, are high in carbohydrates, and have a high osmolality.
4. Avoid the BRAT diet because it is low in energy, proteins, and electrolytes and high in carbohydrates.

IRON-DEFICIENCY ANEMIA

Overview

Anemia is a disorder in which there is less than the normal number of RBCs and/or hemoglobin concentration. Iron-deficiency anemia (IDA) is the most common anemia in children. Factors contributing to IDA include rapid growth rate (as seen in toddlers and adolescents), lack of absorption of iron, blood loss, and inadequate dietary supply of iron. IDA occurs most often in children 9 to 24 months old. It usually is related to the intake of a lot of milk and foods that do not contain supplemental iron. The clinical signs of IDA vary but may include tachycardia, lethargy, irritability, extreme pallor, muscle weakness, shortness of breath, and poor sucking in infants.

Pathophysiology

Iron is necessary for the body to manufacture the hemoglobin (Hgb) in RBCs. When there is not enough iron, the bone marrow continues to produce RBCs but with less Hgb, causing these RBCs to carry oxygen inefficiently, which deprives vital organs of adequate oxygen. This decreases peripheral vascular resistance, which increases cardiac workload, producing the manifestations seen in an anemic state.

IDA is not usually seen prior to 9 months of age because a normal full-term neonate is born with enough stored iron to produce enough Hgb for 4 to 6 months.

Key assessments and rationales

1. Obtain a complete family and neonatal health history and do a physical assessment.
   A health history identifies any deficiencies. A neonatal history is important because the fetus stores iron during the 3rd trimester, so

infants born before 32 weeks require supplemental iron sooner.
2. Assess the child's past and current diet and nutritional status.
   Therapy is based on history. If cow's milk is introduced into the child's diet before he is 12 months old, he does not get the needed iron from iron-fortified formula.
3. Assess for tachycardia, shortness of breath, waxy pallor, lethargy, frequent resting, poor sucking, and feeding.
   These are manifestations of anemia.

Key interventions and rationales
1. Prepare the child and parents for diagnostic blood tests.
   Measuring hemoglobin, iron-binding capacity, and ferritin levels are done to confirm disorder. Having the parents and child know what to expect relieves anxiety and fear.
2. Encourage the parents to stay with the child as much as possible.
   This helps minimize separation anxiety.
3. Take the child's vital signs during periods of activity and rest.
   This provides data for comparison during the periods.
4. Maintain the child in a high Fowler's position.
   This position best promotes optimal air exchange.
5. Observe the child for signs of physical exertion.
   This provides data to plan rest periods and to prevent unnecessary exertion.
6. Anticipate and assist in ADLs that may be beyond the child's tolerance.
   Children with IDA can tire easily and may not be able to complete their hygiene activities.

Drugs commonly used in this disorder
1. Ferrous sulfate--this oral iron supplement prevents and treats IDA. It aids in the formation of Hgb. Dose range: 3 to 6 mg/kg/24 hours PO in one dose or two divided doses. Nursing considerations include administering iron before meals; avoiding giving with milk, eggs, or antacids as they decrease absorption; giving with vitamin C rich foods, such as orange juice, as these increase the absorption of iron in the body; administering liquid iron through a straw, medicine dropper, or brush or wipe off teeth to minimize teeth staining; and advising parents that black tarry stools indicates an adequate dose of iron.

Nutrition considerations
1. Provide iron-fortified formula or breast feed until child is 12 months old.
2. For the child over 12 months old, limit cow's milk to 24 ounces a day or less, as it is not rich in iron.
3. Increase the child's intake of iron-rich foods with selections based on age and developmental level.

ACETAMINOPHEN POISONING

Overview
Accidental poisoning in young children is a serious public health problem. Toddlers, because of their developmental characteristics of curiosity and activity, are prone to ingest substances that can be potentially fatal. While many household substances are ingested accidentally, acetaminophen (Tylenol) is the most common drug causing accidental poisoning in children. Other foreign substances children ingest include cleansers, oil-based products like gasoline, cosmetics, perfumes, aftershave, diaper care products, and vitamins. In many cases, other common medications found in the home, such as oral contraceptives, cough medicine, and antibiotics, cause accidental poisoning.

The nurse's role in accidental poisoning is to assess and treat the child. Interventions to assure support of vital functions is a primary concern. Determining what was ingested, how much, and when, and help determine the treatment protocol.

Pathophysiology
A metabolite of acetaminophen damages the liver. Glutathione, a normally present liver enzyme, neutralizes the acetaminophen metabolite, which is then excreted in the urine. When high doses of acetaminophen are ingested, the metabolite overwhelms the neutralization process, causing hepatic necrosis.

Key assessments and rationales
1. Take the child's vital signs and do a physical assessment.
   The most important rule in treating accidental poisoning is to treat the child and not the poison. Immediate concern for the potential need for life support must be determined.
2. Assess acetaminophen serum levels.
   As the initial symptoms of acetaminophen poisoning are mild, diagnosis must be confirmed by serum acetaminophen levels.

Levels are determined 4 hours after ingestion and several times thereafter for 24 hours.
3. Ask the parents when and how much of the drug was taken.
Parents or caretakers may be able to give important information about time of ingestion and amount of drug taken.
4. Ask the parents if the child has any childhood disease in progress.
Any mild clinical signs can be confused with those of common child diseases.
5. Ask the parents what home treatment was done.
Knowing what, if any, treatment was done at home guides subsequent treatment decisions.

Key interventions and rationales
1. Give the child prescribed ipecac followed with activated charcoal or gastric lavage to remove the acetaminophen from the stomach.
Since the time of ingestion may not be known, efforts to rid the stomach of any drug should be instituted immediately. The administration of activated charcoal will absorb any remaining drug in the stomach.
2. Give the child n-acetylcysteine as ordered via nasogastric tube.
Giving n-acetylcysteine via nasal tube is less unpleasant. The drug smells like rotten eggs, so many children refuse to take it; it may be diluted in fruit juice or soda.
3. Monitor the child's I&O and fluid balance.
Fluid loss from vomiting may reduce urine output. Liver failure can cause fluid retention as well as reducing urine output.
4. Monitor the child's activity level.
Any slowing in level of activity and level of consciousness can indicate impending hepatic coma.
5. Reassure the parents about the child's condition.
Many parents feel guilty about an accident and will need emotional support and reassurance about their child's condition.
6. Let the parents ventilate their feelings about the accidental poisoning.
Letting them express their feelings about the accident will help resolve any guilt and refocus their attention on their child's health.
7. Teach parents poison-prevention techniques. Recommend that 30 ml (1 ounce) of ipecac syrup be kept available in the home after the child reaches age 1.
Teaching poison-control measures prevent future accidents. Many parents underestimate their children's physical ability and curiosity. Specific guidelines should be taught, such as keeping medications in a tight child-proof container to keep potential poisons out of reach of small children and knowing emergency measures to take if an accident occurs. Poison Control Center telephone numbers should be handy.

Drugs commonly used in this disorder
1. Acetylcysteine (Mucomyst)--this mucolytic helps liquefy respiratory secretions and restores liver glutathione levels to treat Tylenol poisoning. Dose range: 140 mg/kg initially, then 70 mg/kg q4h until 1,330 mg/kg are given. Nursing considerations include starting drug immediately when treating acetaminophen poisoning; diluting with fruit juice if giving orally; and repeating dose if child vomits within 1 hour of receiving a dose.
2. Ipecac syrup--this stimulates vomiting by local action on the gastric lining. Dose range: 6 to 12 months, 10 ml followed by 100 to 200 ml of water. Do not repeat. Emesis of children at home is contraindicated between 6 and 10 months of age. Ipecac should be administered only in a health care facility because of risk of aspiration. Ages 1 to 12 years, 15 ml followed by 200 ml of water or milk. Repeat dose once if vomiting has not occurred in 20 minutes. Over 12 years, 15 to 30 ml followed by 200 to 300 ml of water. Repeat dose once if vomiting has not occurred in 20 minutes. Nursing considerations include observing for 1 hour (the drug works in 20 or 30 minutes). Do not give if signs of shock or child is semi-comatose; also do not give if petroleum products have been ingested.

Nutrition considerations
1. NPO until ipecac and acetylcysteine therapy are completed.
2. Liquids to regular diet as tolerated.

<table>
<tr><td colspan="3">STAGES OF ACUTE ACETAMINOPHEN POISONING</td></tr>
<tr><td colspan="3">The stages of acute acetaminophen poisoning are outlined here. During the first stage, acute illness develops and is followed by a subclinical progression of hepatic damage, resulting in later abnormal laboratory findings and the return of clinical findings. The last stage represents possible long-term outcomes from the poisoning.</td></tr>
<tr><td>Stage</td><td>Onset</td><td>Signs and symptoms</td></tr>
<tr><td>I</td><td>1 to 24 hours after ingestion. Initial period is usually 2 to 4 hours after ingestion.</td><td>Anorexia, nausea, vomiting, malaise, pallor, diaphoresis</td></tr>
<tr><td>II</td><td>24 to 48 hours after ingestion</td><td><ul><li>Latency period, with resolution Stage I signs and symptoms</li><li>Early manifestations of subclinical hepatic dysfunction, such as right upper quadrant pain and tenderness, oliguria, elevated serum bilirubin level, increased prothrombin time, and increased hepatic enzyme levels</li></ul></td></tr>
<tr><td>III</td><td>72 to 96 hours after ingestion</td><td><ul><li>Peak liver function abnormalities</li><li>Possible reappearance of Stage I signs and symptoms</li></ul></td></tr>
<tr><td>IV</td><td>4 days to 2 weeks after ingestion</td><td><ul><li>Beginning of resolution of hepatic dysfunction (full hepatic recovery may take 3 months)</li><li>Possible complications: disseminated intravascular coagulation, renal failure, pancreatitis</li></ul></td></tr>
</table>

TETRALOGY OF FALLOT

Overview

Tetralogy of Fallot (TOF) is the most common cyanotic cardiac defect, accounting for 9% to 10% of all congenital heart defects. TOF is named for a French physician who identified four specific cardiac abnormalities that occur simultaneously: (1) ventricular septal defect (VSD); (2) pulmonic stenosis; (3) overriding of the aorta; and (4) right ventricular hypertrophy.

TOF is a defect of decreased pulmonary blood flow. Blood has difficulty exiting the right side of the heart via the pulmonary artery because of the stenosis; thus pressure on the right side increases, eventually exceeding left-sided pressure. This lets desaturated blood shunt right to left, causing desaturation in the left side of the heart and in the systemic circulation. Clinically, these infants are hypoxemic and usually appear cyanotic.

In most cases, complete repair of the defect is performed in the first year of life and involves closure of the VSD, pulmonary valvotomy and enlargement of the right ventricular outflow tract.

Pathophysiology
TOF occurs as a result of abnormal fetal development. The area where the pulmonary artery should emanate develops abnormally, prohibiting the outflow of blood from the heart. The lungs may be supplied with blood because of collateral circulation from the aorta. An improper alignment of embryonic tissue causes a large VSD, displacing the aorta so that it lies directly over the ventricular septum. Right ventricular hypertrophy develops as a direct consequence to the increased workload that occurs with pulmonary stenosis.

When the pulmonary stenosis is mild, the right ventricular pressure is slightly elevated, and there is minimal shunting of blood through the VSD. When pulmonary blood flow is severely obstructed, a lot of venous blood is shunted through the VSD from the right ventricle into the aorta, producing arterial oxygen desaturation. The more severe the stenosis, the greater the right-to-left shunt through the VSD. Unoxygenated blood bypasses the lungs and enters the aorta directly, mixing oxygenated blood with unoxygenated blood in systemic circulation, causing hypoxemia.

Key assessments and rationales
1. Assess the infant for cyanosis, tachycardia, dyspnea (during or after feeding), failure to thrive, respiratory distress, exercise intolerance, clubbing of digits, and squatting episodes.
   These are clinical manifestations, physical consequences, and compensatory mechanisms of TOF.
2. Assess the infant's height and weight and plot on a growth chart.
   This will determine growth trend. Infants with congenital heart defects may demonstrate a failure to thrive and growth retardation.

3. Assess the infant's behavior during feedings.
   Many infants with heart disease need to pause frequently during feedings, have a poor sucking reflex, and have difficulty coordinating sucking, swallowing, and breathing. Anoxic spells may occur during feedings.
4. Assess the infant's chest contours.
   A raised sternum indicates the presence of right ventricular hypertrophy.

Key interventions and rationales
1. Obtain baseline vital sign parameters for each infant. Set cardiopulmonary monitor limits accordingly and monitor q2-4h.
   Infants with congestive heart failure will experience changes in their vital signs because of increased at-rest fluid retention. Baseline vital signs and monitoring will help determine changes in their status. Actual findings may fall outside the range of expected norms.
2. Monitor the infant's respiratory status every 1 or 2 hours, assessing rate, chest expansion, use of accessory muscles, nasal flaring, grunting, retractions, and auscultation of breath sounds.
   Early signs of inadequate gas exchange are exhibited by respiratory difficulty. Pulmonary edema develops rapidly and, in fragile infants, can be manifested by decreased breath sounds.
3. Elevate the infant's head and upper body to facilitate respiratory effort and decrease the work of breathing.
   Elevating the head and upper body promotes the shift of fluid from the lungs, so less respiratory effort is required.
4. Administer humidified oxygen during times of exertion and stress.
   An increase in the blood-oxygen level helps decrease the need for greater cardiac output.
5. Keep the infant free of stress by meeting his feeding and comfort needs promptly.
   Crying and agitation may precipitate hypercyanotic episodes.
6. Monitor the infant for hypercyanosis. If it occurs, place him in knee-chest position and notify his health care provider.
   Severe hypercyanotic episodes can cause metabolic acidosis, syncope, seizures, cerebral vascular accident (CVA), unconsciousness, and death. The lateral knee-chest position increases pulmonary blood flow by increasing systemic vascular resistance. This improves systemic arterial oxygen saturation by decreasing venous return, so less highly saturated blood reaches the heart.
7. Monitor the infant for signs of increasing heart failure.

Worsening heart failure can progress rapidly. Signs are peripheral edema, trunk, head, and neck edema.

8. Check the infant's weight q12-24h, I&O hourly, and urine specific gravity 4 to 6 times a day.
   Infants with heart failure will urinate less because of fluid retention. An imbalance between I&O is significant because it provides information as to how much fluid is being retained. Weight gain may indicate fluid retention.

9. Palpate the liver once a shift.
   An increase in liver size may indicate right-sided heart failure.

10. Explain the disorder to the parents and encourage them to spend time with their infant and participate as much as possible in his care.
    Explanations can ease anxiety; participation lets parents maintain their role, eases their sense of loss of control, and lets them support their infant.

Drugs commonly used in this disorder

1. Digoxin (Lanoxin)--this digitalis glycoside slows the heart rate, increases the force and velocity of contractions, increases cardiac output, slows atrioventricular conduction, and indirectly enhances diuresis by increasing renal perfusion. Dose range depends on age and weight. Infants usually are digitalized with a loading dose and maintained on daily dose, never exceeding 0.25 mg/kg/day. Nursing considerations include measuring apical rate and rhythm for 1 full minute; monitoring I&O and taking daily weights; assessing serum electrolytes, especially potassium; being alert for signs of digoxin toxicity. Do not mix I.V. digoxin with other drugs; if child vomits, do not give a second dose but notify health care provider. Do not mix PO digoxin with food or fluids.

2. Alprostadil (Prostaglandin E1: PGE1)--this vasodilator is used in neonates only if closure of the ductus arteriosus causes life-threatening cyanosis. PGE1 is a palliative medication and is prescribed to reopen or maintain the ductus arteriosus. Dose range: initial dosage for neonates is 0.05 to 0.1 mcg/kg/minute and may advance to 0.2 mcg/kg/minute if necessary. Nursing considerations include taking baseline vital signs and monitoring vital signs; and maintaining the infant on cardiopulmonary monitor. Use cautiously in infants with bleeding tendencies.

Nutrition considerations

1. Provide small frequent feedings with adequate protein and calories

to promote growth.

2. Infants with heart failure usually are placed on a diet consisting of no added salt. Sodium-restricted or salt-free diets are not used in children because of their potential negative effects on their appetite and ultimate growth.

3. Provide potassium-rich foods or potassium supplements if infant is on a diuretic. Mix the elixir with fruit juice to disguise the bitter taste and to prevent intestinal irritation from a concentrated solution.

OTITIS MEDIA

Overview

Otitis media (OM) is an inflammation of the mucosal lining of the middle ear characterized by a rapid onset of symptoms lasting approximately 3 weeks. The disorder is one of the most common illnesses of childhood and is most prevalent between 6 months and 3 years of age, gradually decreasing with age. It is rare in children over 7 years old.

The incidence is highest in the winter months and in children living in households with smokers. Complications include conductive hearing loss, mastoiditis, meningitis, brain abscess, and perforation of the tympanic membrane.

Pathophysiology

A young child's eustachian tubes are short, wide, and straight; they lie in a relatively straight plane. The cartilage lining is underdeveloped, making the tubes easily distended and thus more likely to open inappropriately, letting pathogens enter. The young child's normally large pharyngeal tissue easily obstructs the eustachian tube openings in the nasopharynx, impairing drainage, and an infant's supine position favors the pooling of fluid in the pharyngeal cavity.

When the eustachian tube is blocked because of enlarged adenoids or mucosal edema from an upper respiratory infection, adequate drainage and ventilation of the middle ear cannot occur. Air, normally present in the middle ear, is absorbed by the blood, resulting in negative pressure and fluid (effusion) accumulating within the middle ear, supplying a medium for bacterial growth. When an infection occurs, purulent fluid accumulates in the middle ear space, causing pressure and pain.

Key assessments and rationales

1. Assess if child has had a recent upper respiratory infection (URI).
   URI often precedes an episode of OM.
2. Assess the child for fever, ear pain (head rolling and pulling at the ear), and postauricular and cervical lymph gland enlargement.
   These are clinical manifestations of OM.
3. Examine the child's ear, inspecting the tympanic membrane with an otoscope. Note color, mobility, and translucency.
   Evaluate the tympanic membrane and identify any perforation of the eardrum.
4. Observe for ear drainage, noting its color, consistency, and odor. Send for culture and sensitivity.
   This will help diagnose bacterial, viral, or allergy-caused OM.
5. Assess the child's hearing and language development.
   Evaluate any hearing loss or impairment.

Key interventions and rationales

1. Administer analgesics and antipyretics.
   This will reduce pain and fever.
2. Apply heating pad on low setting, wrapped in a towel, over the child's ear as he lies on his affected side.
   This will promote comfort and ear drainage.
3. Apply an ice pack over the affected ear.
   This helps reduce edema and ear pressure.
4. Teach the parents the importance of adhering to a regular drug schedule and completing the course of antibiotic therapy.
   This will prevent recurrence of infection.
5. Teach gentle nose blowing while a URI is present.
   This will decrease the risk of transferring organisms from the eustachian tube to the middle ear.
6. Advise parents not to expose child to cigarette smoke.
   Passive smoke increases the incidence of OM.
7. Stress the importance of follow-up flu care.
   This will ensure that the ear is free of infection and effusion and that the child's hearing is normal.

Drugs commonly used in this disorder

1. Amoxicillin/clavulanate potassium (Augmentin)--this bactericidal antibiotic inhibits bacterial wall synthesis by adhering to bacterial penicillin-binding proteins. Dose range: 20 to 40 mg/kg/24 hours divided q8h for 10 days. Nursing considerations include assessing

history of hypersensitivity; monitoring renal function; administering at least 1 hour before bacteriostatic antibiotics; giving drug with meals if GI distress occurs; maintaining fluid intake; shaking suspension well; and observing for signs of superinfection. Tabs may be crushed.

2. Cefaclor (Ceclor)--this second-generation cephalosporin antibiotic inhibits bacterial protein synthesis by adhering to penicillin-binding enzymes. Dose range: 20 mg/kg/24 hours in divided doses q8-12h. Nursing considerations are the same as for Augmentin, plus monitoring for signs of bleeding because of prolonged bleeding time.

Nutrition considerations
1. Offer liquids or soft foods to avoid chewing.
2. Hold or sit infant upright for feedings to prevent pooling of formula in the pharyngeal cavity.

TYPE 1 DIABETES MELLITUS

Overview
Type 1 diabetes mellitus (DM) is the most common metabolic disease in children. It is an autoimmune process that destroys the insulin-secreting cells in the pancreas. Genetics, autoimmunity, diet, viruses, and environmental factors have all been linked to the destruction of beta cells. The primary features of diabetes include hyperglycemia; abnormalities in carbohydrate, protein, and fat metabolism; and an increased incidence of eye, renal, neurologic, and premature cardiovascular diseases. The peak incidence of the disorder is between 10 and 14 years of age. Successful management of diabetes is dependent on the family's and child's commitment to a regimen that includes monitoring blood glucose levels with day-to-day adjustment of insulin, and adherence to a diet and exercise program.

Pathophysiology
Glucose is the primary source of energy for all body cells. It is derived from dietary sources and is produced and stored in the liver and muscles as glycogen. Glucose homeostasis is regulated by the interaction of several hormones, including insulin and glucagon. Both hormones are secreted directly into the bloodstream in response to changes in the plasma glucose concentration. The primary function of insulin is to regulate blood glucose levels by controlling the rate at which blood glucose is utilized by the body.

Type 1 DM occurs when the pancreas is unable to produce and secrete insulin. In the absence of insulin, the metabolism of fats, proteins, and carbohydrates is impaired. Glucose is unable to move into the cells, resulting in hyperglycemia. As blood glucose levels surpass the renal threshold, glucose spills into the urine, causing polyuria. Polydipsia follows in response to the fluid loss. Fatigue, hunger, and weight loss seen in uncontrolled diabetes result from cellular starvation from the absence of insulin. Ketones, manufactured by the liver from adipose tissue, are produced in response to cellular starvation. In the absence of insulin, ketones are unavailable to the cell for sustenance. Increasing blood levels of ketones eventually result in ketoacidosis.

Key assessments and rationales

1. Obtain a thorough health history and perform a physical exam.
   Find out whether onset of signs and symptoms were preceded by an infectious illness, if there is a family history, and estimate the severity of metabolic alteration.
2. Assess for polyuria, polydipsia and polyphagia, and significant weight loss.
   These are cardinal, classic symptoms of DM and hyperglycemia.
3. Assess medications currently being used.
   Glucocorticoids and some chemotherapeutic agents can cause hyperglycemia.
4. Assess for dry mucous membranes, flushed skin, absence of tearing, and poor skin turgor.
   These are signs and symptoms of dehydration associated with polyuria.
5. Assess for recurrent vaginal and urinary tract infections, especially candida infection.
   These are often early signs of diabetes, especially in adolescents.
6. Assess for abdominal pain, nausea, vomiting, Kussmaul's respirations, fruity breath, and changes in the level of consciousness.
   These are signs and symptoms of ketoacidosis.
7. Assess the family's knowledge of diabetes and their learning ability.
   This will help you prepare for future teaching. Determining the family's understanding of the disorder is essential because misinformation is common.
8. Assess the family's ability to cope with a chronic illness and identify their usual methods of coping with stress.
   Determine what interventions and referrals may be needed.

Key interventions and rationales

1. Monitor the child's I&O and weight daily.
   This will determine hydration status. Dehydration is present to some extent in uncontrolled diabetes.
2. Maintain fluid and electrolyte replacement.
   Correct replacement is essential to achieving metabolic stability.
3. Monitor blood glucose level as ordered.
   This will determine the most appropriate dose of insulin.
4. Test for urinary ketones when the blood glucose is over 250 mg/dl or when the child is sick.
   Ketones are formed in response to an insulin deficit and are often present with high glucose values or an illness.
5. Teach the parents how to recognize the signs of hypoglycemia early and what to do if it occurs.
   Hypoglycemia is a potentially dangerous state. Knowing the signs and interventions can avert a serious problem.
6. Teach the child and family the characteristics of the prescribed insulin, storage and care of insulin and equipment, correct mixing of insulin, injection procedure, and rotational sites.
   This will ensure proper diabetic management at home.
7. Teach the child and family urine ketone testing and blood glucose monitoring and the interpretation of results.
   They need to learn how to adjust insulin based on blood glucose level.
8. Encourage daily exercise.
   Exercise is an important factor in lowering blood glucose levels. It increases the body's sensitivity to insulin and decreases serum cholesterol and triglyceride levels, thereby lowering the risk of developing cardiovascular complications.
9. Emphasize the importance of personal hygiene and proper care of cuts and abrasions.
   This will minimize the risk of infection.
10. Advise the child to wear a medic-alert bracelet.
    In case of an emergency, caregivers need to know the child has diabetes.
11. Identify community support systems available for the child and family, such as age-specific support groups, parent support group, and diabetes summer camp.
    Community resources are an excellent source of information and emotional support, and they are an alternative to relying solely on family coping skills.

Drugs commonly used in this disorder

1. Insulin--this pancreatic hormone enables glucose transport across cell membranes to reduce blood glucose. Insulin must be administered subcutaneously or intravenously. Dose range is

individualized, depending on blood glucose levels. Nursing considerations include assessing for manifestations of hyperglycemia or hypoglycemia; assessing blood glucose and urine ketones; and teaching the child and family how store and how to prepare insulin for administration and site rotation. Always draw up short-acting insulin before long-acting insulin. Tell the parents that the child should carry simple sugar (hard candy) at all times and wear a medic-alert device.

Nutrition considerations
1. Follow diabetic diet planned by dietician. Caloric intake is determined by the child's needs.
2. Balance food intake with the amount of insulin being taken.
3. Eliminate concentrated sweets.
4. Reduce fat to 30% or less of total caloric requirement because of increased risk for atherosclerosis.
5. Dietary fiber influences the digestion, absorption, and metabolism of many nutrients and can diminish the rise in blood glucose after meals.

CYSTIC FIBROSIS

Overview
Cystic fibrosis (CF) is a chronic, multisystem, heredity disorder of the exocrine glands, affecting the airways, pancreas, intestinal tract, and sweat glands. The mucus produced by the exocrine glands is abnormally thick, obstructing the small passageways of various organs. CF ranks as the leading fatal genetic illness among Caucasians. It is inherited as an autosomal recessive trait.

Although CF is incurable, aggressive chest physiotherapy, aerosol treatments, antibiotics, nutritional education, and advances in protein and gene therapy improve the life expectancy in affected children dramatically. The median survival age is 30 years.

Pathophysiology
The respiratory system pathology is the most significant aspect of CF, ultimately accounting for the morbidity and 90% of the mortality.

The bronchial mucous glands produce a lot of thick, dry mucus. This along with abnormalities in ciliary motility leads to chronic secretion retention, producing diffuse airway obstruction, increasing airway resistance, and contributing to areas of atelectasis. Secretion retention leads to chronic gram-positive and gram-negative bacterial colonization and recurrent infection.

The presence of secretions in the airways can contribute to the development of bronchiectasis, which leads to obstructive pulmonary disease. Chronic hypoxemia leads to increased pulmonary vascular resistance (PVR), pulmonary hypertension, and eventually cor pulmonale. Nutritional abnormalities occur secondary to dysfunction of the pancreas and intestine. The pancreatic ducts, blocked by thick mucus, are unable to secrete trypsin, amylase, and lipase into the small intestine. Without these digestive enzymes, proteins, carbohydrates, and fats are poorly absorbed.

Key assessments and rationales
1. Perform a physical assessment, plot height and weight on a standardized growth chart.
   Obtain baseline information and assess developmental level.
2. Obtain a complete health history.
   Many children with CF have frequent episodes of bronchopneumonia and bronchitis. A diet history reveals caloric intake, use of pancreatic enzymes, and vitamins.
3. Auscultate the child's chest to detect any crackles, wheezes, areas of diminished breath sounds, or prolonged expiratory phase of respiration.
   These indicate pulmonary involvement.
4. Assess rate, depth, ease of respirations, dyspnea, cyanosis, color of nail beds and mucous membranes, and pulse oximetry values.
   This helps determine the degree of respiratory distress.
5. Assess the characteristics of the child's cough and the color, amount, and quality of sputum.
   This helps determine whether an infection is present.
6. Assess the child's exercise tolerance and ability to sleep lying down.
   Determining the level of any physical limitations helps plan for care.
7. Auscultate bowel sounds and assess for abdominal pain, blood in the stools, and constipation.
   Assess for ulcers and intestinal obstruction that often accompany CF.
8. Assess for steatorrhea, frequent infections, fatigue, and protuberant abdomen.
   These indicate malabsorption.
9. Assess the child's immunization status.
   Children with CF should get all routine immunizations, in addition to the annual influenza vaccine by the Centers for Disease Control and Prevention (CDC).

Key interventions and rationales

1. Monitor the child's vital signs and pulse oximetry readings.
   This will help detect and prevent hypoxemia.
2. Administer humidified supplemental oxygen, if ordered, and monitor the child closely.
   Oxygen-induced carbon dioxide narcosis is an oxygen therapy hazard in any client with chronic pulmonary disease.
3. Elevate the head of the bed or support the child in an upright position with pillows if he is dyspneic.
   An upright position facilitates chest expansion by decreasing pressure on the diaphragm.
4. During an acute exacerbation, organize daily activities and nursing care to allow for rest periods.
   This permits minimum expenditure of the child's energy.
5. Help the child expectorate mucus, using nebulization, chest physiotherapy, and suction, if necessary.
   This promotes airway clearance, facilitates lung expansion, and liquefies, and loosens and clears secretions.
6. Administer fluids, PO or I.V.
   Adequate fluid intake decreases the viscosity of secretions and aids in expectoration.
7. Provide frequent mouth care, especially before meals and snacks.
   Copious, tenacious sputum produces a foul taste and decreases appetite.
8. Observe frequency and nature of stools.
   Fewer, less fatty and less foul-smelling stools indicate adequate enzyme replacement.
9. Encourage physical activity, as tolerated.
   Exercise is often effective in clearing accumulated pulmonary secretions.
10. Encourage the child to express his feelings about the illness. Help him identify personal strengths and areas of accomplishments.
    The physical changes with CF may affect self-worth. Recognition and pride in special attributes increases self-esteem.
11. Encourage the child to participate in and take responsibility for self-care as much as possible.
    Active participation in decision-making promotes autonomy and adherence to the treatment plan.
12. Provide information about resources, such as the Cystic Fibrosis Foundation, American Lung Association, and Crippled Children's programs.

Help the family get information, equipment, and financial support that will help them cope with the stresses of a chronic illness.

Drugs commonly used in this disorder

1. Acetylcysteine (Mucomyst)--this mucolytic agent decreases the viscosity of secretions by breaking disulfide links of mucoproteins. It is indicated for use as an adjunctive therapy in children with abnormal or thick mucous secretions accompanying acute or chronic pulmonary disease. Dose range: for infants is 1 to 2 ml 20% solution or 2 to 4 ml 10% solution via nebulizer t.i.d. to q.i.d.; for children, the dose is 3 to 5 ml 20% solution or 6 to 10 ml 10% solution via nebulizer t.i.d. to q.i.d.; for adolescents, the dose is 5 to 10 ml 10% to 20% solution via nebulizer t.i.d. to q.i.d. Nursing considerations include assessing vital signs, cardiac rhythm, pulse oximeter, and breath sounds before and after treatment; discontinuing treatment if bronchospasm occurs; and rinsing mouth after nebulizer treatment.
2. Recombinant human deoxyribonuclease 1 (rhDNase)--this drug cleaves DNA in the purulent sputum, reducing viscosity and enhancing secretion clearance. The dosing schedule may involve inhalation three times a day, 5 days a week, for 2 weeks. It is well tolerated and has no major adverse effects.

Nutrition considerations

1. Feed infants predigested or partially digested formulas, such as Pregestimil, Portagen and Nutramigen. Encourage breast-feeding.
2. Because of malabsorption and the stress of illness, older children require 150% of the normal protein and caloric requirements to maintain growth. Include the client's favorite foods in the diet.
3. Administer pancreatic enzymes within 30 minutes of eating meals and snacks, since replacement of enzymes is necessary for digestion to occur.
4. Provide adequate salt, especially when sweating (from fever, hot weather, physical exertion) since abnormally high sodium and chloride concentrations in the sweat predispose the child to rapid loss of these electrolytes.
5. Let older children take enteric-coated pancreatic enzyme capsules; they must not be crushed or chewed, as this would inactivate the enzymes and excoriate the oral mucosa.
6. Administer fat-soluble multivitamins in water miscible form because impaired digestion and absorption of fat decreases the uptake of the fat-soluble vitamins A, D, E, and K.

CRITICAL THINKING EXERCISE

Pediatric Nursing

Facts and objectives
1. The NCLEX-RN tests your ability to make sound clinical judgments.
2. Developing critical thinking skills is the foundation for being able to make good clinical judgments.
3. This exercise will help you evaluate how well you think critically.
4. As you work through this exercise, you will learn how the continuous flow of questions that evolve as you think the case through will lead you to reach solid conclusions about the client problem and the *best* nursing behaviors.

Instructions
Respond to the following questions by writing down your best thoughts, ideas and "answers." Do this for all of the questions, then turn the page to see what you should have considered in response to each question.

Naturally, to learn to think critically, don't look for hints or answers before completing all questions...don't cheat yourself! How you answer the critical questions will depend on how well you perfect your thinking skills.

ASTHMA
Overview
Jennifer, age 14, is brought to the emergency department by her mother. Jennifer has had asthma or RAD since age 3 and has had numerous hospitalizations. This episode began with a dry cough and slight expiratory wheezing 1 day ago and now has progressed to a severe attack. On auscultation, Jennifer has decreased breath sounds and a prolonged expiratory wheeze.

1. Discuss the factors that can precipitate or aggravate an asthmatic episode.

2. On initial appraisal, what clinical manifestations would the nurse typically assess in a child with an asthma episode? What clinical manifestations are ominous signs and what do they indicate?

3. Describe the therapeutic management, nursing assessments, and interventions that should be provided Jennifer on arrival to the emergency department. What are the rationales for these?

4. Jennifer fails to improve and is admitted to the hospital and begun on theophylline (Aminophylline) via an I.V. infusion pump. Discuss the action of theophylline, signs and symptoms of toxicity, and nursing implications. Since theophylline is now considered a third-line agent for treating asthma, what circumstances would cause it to be prescribed?

5. On discharge, what strategies can the nurse teach Jennifer and her family to help reduce the incidence of Jennifer's acute asthma episodes?

6. Upon discharge, Jennifer is given prescription for Cromolyn sodium (Intal). What is the action of Cromolyn sodium and what information should Jennifer and her parents get about the use of this drug?

7. Discuss age-appropriate self-management of asthma for Jennifer.

THE FOLLOWING ARE INTERVENTIONS AND NURSING BEHAVIORS YOU SHOULD HAVE CONSIDERED IN ANSWERING THE PREVIOUS QUESTIONS.

1. **Discuss the factors that can precipitate or aggravate an asthmatic episode.**
    * *Allergens--foods, animal dander, mold spores, pollens, dust mites, insects, infesting agents, drugs*
    * *Irritants--paint odors, hair sprays, perfumes, chemicals, air pollutants, active and passive smoke, cold air, cold water*
    * *Weather changes*
    * *Infections*
    * *Exercise that is overly vigorous, strenuous, and associated with breathlessness*
    * *Emotional factors--however, there is no evidence that psychologic factors are the basis for asthma*
    * *Gastroesophageal reflux--considered a cause of nocturnal asthma*
    * *Allergic rhinitis, sinusitis, and URI*
    * *Non-allergic hypersensitivity to drugs and chemicals*
    * *Endocrine factors--menstrual cycle, birth-control pills, hyperthyroidism*

2. **On initial appraisal, what clinical manifestations would the nurse typically assess in a child with an asthma episode? What clinical manifestations are ominous signs and what do they indicate?**

    Assessment findings:
    * *Wheezing may be worse at night; may be sudden or gradual and is often preceded by rhinorrhea*
    * *Dyspnea with prolonged expiration and use of accessory muscles of respiration; may also display subclavicular and intercostal retractions, nasal flaring, or stridor*
    * *Non-productive cough (with or without wheezing); later becomes productive; vomiting may accompany the effort of severe coughing*
    * *Tachypnea, orthopnea, dehydration (because of vomiting and tachypnea)*
    * *Restlessness, apprehension, diaphoresis, pallor (as oxygen saturation levels drop)*
    * *Abdominal pain, secondary to the strain placed on stomach muscles during labored breathing*
    * *A "hunched over" sitting position with arms braced, using all accessory muscles for respiration*
    * *Fatigue, as evidenced by difficulty performing simple tasks because of shortness of breath*
    * *Feeling of chest tightness, followed by dry cough, wheezing, and dyspnea*

    Ominous signs:
    * *Decreased wheezing in a child who otherwise is not improving clinically may be incorrectly interpreted as a positive sign when, in fact, it may signal an inability to move air, an obstruction, fatigue, and respiratory failure; a "silent chest" is an ominous sign during an asthma episode*

- *Shortness of breath with air movement in the chest restricted to the point of absent breath sounds*
- *Sudden rise in respiratory rate indicating ventilatory failure and imminent asphyxia*

3. **Describe the therapeutic management, nursing assessments and interventions that should be provided Jennifer on arrival to the emergency department. What are the rationales for these?**
    - *Provide a calm, relaxed, supportive atmosphere; encouragement and support can diminish the anxiety-related increase in oxygen consumption. Calmly present questions and focus on precipitating factors, duration of the attack, course of previous episodes, medications taken, and known allergies.*
    - *Administer humidified oxygen either by nasal prongs or face mask because hypoxemia is a common consequence of airway obstruction. Encourage Jennifer to assume a comfortable position (usually Fowler or semi-Fowler).*
    - *Maintain her on a pulse oximeter and a cardiopulmonary monitor.*
    - *Evaluate her quickly for signs of hypoxemia (headache, anxiety, confusion, dizziness) or impending respiratory failure (drowsiness, diaphoresis, decreased oxygen saturation via pulse oximetry)*
    - *Lung auscultation should be done to evaluate airflow. In severe bronchospasm, no wheezing is audible or it occurs with inspiration--a sign of impending respiratory failure. In less severe episodes, wheezing is heard on both expiration and inspiration. Wheezing that clears with change of position or coughing is caused by mucus that narrows large airways. Frequent chest auscultation for air exchange is critical.*
    - *Arterial blood gases are obtained to assess carbon dioxide and oxygen levels.*
    - *Provide a bronchodilator (beta adrenergics are the medications of choice for the treatment of acute exacerbations of asthma; usually albuterol, terbutaline or metaproterenol) is administered via a power nebulizer. Increased wheezing may be heard after treatment, signaling increased air movement.*
    - *Evaluate hydration status (urine specific gravity helps establish hydration needs).*
    - *An I.V. line is started for fluid and electrolyte maintenance (serum electrolytes should be used to determine the need for potassium replacement) as well as for venous access for parenteral medications.*
    - *Administer prescribed corticosteroids--these decrease inflammation and edema in the airways and potentiate the action of beta-adrenergic bronchodilators; early administration is necessary because the drug will not take effect for 6 or more hours.*
    - *During emergency care, questions posed to Jennifer should be minimal and limited to those that can be answered "yes" or "no." The parents should be permitted to stay to offer reassurance and comfort.*
    - *Once the attack has diminished enough that Jennifer can swallow without gasping, offer her small but frequent drinks of fluids to help liquefy and bring up secretions.*
    - *Chest physical therapy (CPT) may be ordered to help remove secretions after Jennifer has become stabilized. A bronchodilator should be given prior to CPT and postural drainage; an antibiotic should be given following.*

4. **Jennifer fails to improve and is admitted to the hospital and begun on theophylline (Aminophylline) via an I.V. infusion pump. Discuss the action of theophylline, signs and symptoms of toxicity, and nursing implications. Since theophylline is now considered a third-line agent for treating asthma, what circumstances would cause it to be prescribed?**

- *Theophylline relaxes bronchial smooth muscle, decreases airway reactivity, and inhibits mast cell degranulation. Theophylline can be given orally or parenterally, but aerosol administration is ineffective. I.V. theophylline is used in the treatment of acute asthma episodes.*
- *Theophylline is most therapeutic at serum concentrations of 10 to 20 mcg/ml. The rates of theophylline metabolism are extremely variable among children, and the margin between therapeutic and toxic levels is narrow, so serum theophylline levels are monitored closely.*
- *Theophylline toxicity occurs at serum levels exceeding 20 mcg/ml. Manifestations of toxicity include restlessness, nausea, vomiting, irritability, headache, abdominal pain, diarrhea, fever, cardiac arrhythmias, and seizures.*
- *Theophylline is metabolized in the liver, and many factors affect the clearance, thus affecting the serum levels of the drug.*

Decreased clearance (increased serum level):

a. *viral respiratory infection*
b. *erythromycin*
c. *oral contraceptives*
d. *influenza trivalent vaccine*

e. *high-carbohydrate, low-protein diet*
f. *caffeine*
g. *liver or heart failure*

Increased clearance (decreased serum level):

a. *smoking*
b. *phenobarbital*
c. *dilantin*

d. *charcoal-broiled beef*
e. *high-protein, low-carbohydrate diet*

- *Place Jennifer on a cardiopulmonary monitor (theophylline increases heart rate and force of contractions; high blood levels may lead to tachycardia) and have theophylline serum levels drawn after the loading dose and before the maintenance dosage is begun. Observe her closely for signs of theophylline toxicity, and draw serum levels within 6 hours of dosing and again in 12 to 24 hours.*

Theophylline is now considered a third-line agent, even unnecessary for treating asthma episodes. It is a relatively weak bronchodilator compared with the beta adrenergics. Since asthma is now believed to be an inflammatory condition, other drugs are of greater benefit.

Theophylline is used when there is no response to other inhaled medications and for treating chronic asthma. It is effective for longer periods than beta adrenergics and is also useful for the treatment of nighttime symptoms.

5. **On discharge, what strategies can the nurse teach Jennifer and her family to help them reduce the incidence of Jennifer's acute asthma episodes?**
   - *Children with asthma should be encouraged to learn about their condition. Teaching developmentally appropriate self-management skills to children and families has been shown to be an effective tool for improving control over asthma. Teaching the necessary skills to control and manage asthma symptoms can decrease Jennifer's anxiety during episodes and enable her and her family take appropriate action to control the symptoms of the disease.*
   - *The frequency and severity of asthma episodes will be minimized if Jennifer and her family know:*
   --what triggers of asthma to avoid and other preventive measures, such as allergy proofing the home.
   --the early warning signs of an asthma episode.
   --the correct use of treatment aids (nebulizer, metered-dose inhaler).
   --the proper administration of medications, their names, dose, expected effects, adverse effects, and frequency.
   --written guidelines that include when to increase therapy, when to call the health care provider, when to go to the emergency department.
   --strategies to control fear and panic during asthma episodes. Jennifer can practice abdominal breathing and self-relaxation techniques such as guided imagery, along with taking prescribed bronchodilators or beta-adrenergic treatments.
   --the importance of diet, rest, and exercise to prevent asthma symptoms.
   --to keep immunizations up-to-date to protect her from contagious disease.
   --to schedule regular follow-up appointments.

6. **Upon discharge, Jennifer is given prescription for Cromolyn sodium (Intal). What is the action of Cromolyn sodium and what information should Jennifer and her parents get about the use of this drug?**
   - *Cromolyn sodium (Intal) is an inhaled nonsteroidal anti-inflammatory medication that prevents asthma symptoms by blocking the release of mast cell mediators.*
   - *Cromolyn has no effect on asthma symptoms once they have begun because this drug has no bronchodilating effect.*
   - *Cromolyn is primarily used for maintenance therapy in clients with chronic asthma. It may be used before exercise or exposure to a known allergen to prevent symptoms.*
   - *Cromolyn is available as a dry powder inhalation, as a metered-dose inhaler and as a nebulized solution.*
   - *This medication is most effective against allergen-induced asthma when taken 30 minutes before exposure to the allergen.*
   - *Exercise-induced asthma is best prevented when Cromolyn is inhaled a few minutes before exercise (no more than 1 hour before anticipated exercise). Cromolyn works best when the bronchioles are open; an inhaled adrenergic medication may be prescribed prior to administration to Cromolyn.*

- *Cromolyn is a safe drug and is virtually free of adverse effects. Occasionally, inhalation of Cromolyn will irritate the airways, causing a mild cough. Drinking a few sips of water before and after inhalation usually prevents this problem and minimizes the bad taste of this medication.*
- *Jennifer and her family should be aware that Cromolyn is a preventive medication and is not effective for the relief of asthma symptoms.*
- *Cromolyn should also be given on a 4- to 6-week trial in order to obtain the true benefit, as the response to treatment may become apparent only after 2 or 4 weeks of therapy. Jennifer should be instructed to report any coughing or wheezing after administration of Cromolyn.*

7. **Discuss age-appropriate self-management of asthma with Jennifer.**
    - *This client is an adolescent involved in the developmental task of identity and intimacy versus confusion and isolation. She needs to be involved in the decision-making process about her care. Teach her the following responsibilities:*
    --Plan and take routine medications and treatments.
    --Learn and recognize medication adverse effects.
    --Determine and tell parents when medications need to be refilled.
    --Use a peak flow meter correctly and records measurements.
    --Assess the severity of symptoms and identify symptoms early.
    --Recognize when to contact health care provider and discusses this with parents.
    --Avoid and control factors that make asthma worse, both at home and at school.

CHAPTER 7

VIEW THE PROGRAM *"INTERPRETING ECGs"* BEFORE PROCEEDING. IT IS THE 6TH PROGRAM ON THE VIDEO MODULE.

CARDIOVASCULAR SYSTEM
Myocardial infarction

Overview

Myocardial infarction (MI) is the leading cause of death from coronary artery disease. Myocardial infarction is caused by a reduction in the supply of blood from the coronary arteries to the cardiac muscle tissue. These reductions in blood supply can be caused by arterial atherosclerosis, emboli, or thrombus-related occlusions.

Pathophysiology

When blood flow to the myocardium is interrupted because of infarction, the damaged cardiac cells revert to anaerobic metabolism, increasing lactic acid. Necrotic myocardial cells spill intracellular potassium into the extracellular fluid, causing hyperkalemia, resulting in a decreased ability of the remaining cells to generate electrical impulses. Necrosis in the infarcted area of the heart causes enzymes to be released into the extracellular fluid. The enzymes most specific for the diagnosis of an MI are creatine kinase (CK) and the cardiac-specific troponins. Elevated cardiac enzymes, ECG changes, and chest pain all are relevant factors for the diagnosis of an MI.

Key assessments and rationales

1. Take vital signs, being alert to rapid pulse and low blood pressure.
   Frequently checking vital signs will alert to signs (rapid pulse, low blood pressure) of low cardiac output leading to cardiogenic shock.
2. Assess for typical MI crushing chest pain unrelieved by nitroglycerine.
   MI pain produces a sharper, more severe pain than angina, often described as heavy pressure, squeezing, or a heavy dull ache. It is not relieved by nitroglycerine.
3. Obtain and assess a 12-lead ECG, as ordered.
   ECG tracings record ischemia during pain episodes and manifest electrical impulse changes associated with MI.
4. Assess serum enzyme changes, especially isolated MB-bands of the CK, cardiac-specific troponin T and I, and lactic dehydrogenase (LDH) levels.
   Laboratory data help determine cardiac cell death, quantify the

amount of damage, and determine, by changes in peaks and duration, when the MI occurred.

5. Determine the client's support system, level of anxiety, and knowledge of the condition.
A client with an MI is in a life-threatening state. Anxiety increases sympathetic nervous system activity, which increases cardiac workload. Emotional support from family and friends is crucial. Knowledge assessment is important in developing intervention plans to reduce client and family anxiety.

Key interventions and rationales

1. Relieve pain and maintain oxygenation.
Pain relief has priority over all other interventions. Pain makes the heart work harder, increasing cardiac ischemia. Oxygen provides greater blood oxygen saturation in the myocardium, reducing ischemia.
2. Maintain continuous cardiac monitoring.
MI clients are at risk for ventricular arrhythmias leading to fibrillation and conduction defects leading to heart block.
3. Monitor hemodynamics and I&O hourly.
Fluid balance must be maintained to avoid overloading the heart with fluids. Edema, jugular vein distention, and an S3 or S4 are signs of fluid overload and impending failure.
4. Prevent immobility complications.
Change client's position often to decrease immobility problems.
5. Teach the client to avoid Valsalva maneuver.
Valsalva maneuver increases intrathoracic pressure, which decreases blood flow to the heart. The client should not hold his breath while turning in bed. Stool softeners will help prevent straining at stool.
6. Provide an environment that promotes physical and mental rest.
Rest is essential to reduce workload on the heart.
7. Teach the client about antiplatelet and diet therapy, stress testing, and home drug regimen.
Clients need to understand the reason for drug therapy to enhance compliance. Dietary changes may be necessary for long-term cardiac rehabilitation.
8. Assist the client with rehabilitation and lifestyle modifications.
The client will begin a graduated exercise program to improve physical conditioning and cardiac efficiency.

Drugs commonly used in this disorder

1. Morphine sulfate--this opiate narcotic decreases pain perception by acting on the opiate receptors in the CNS. Dose range: 4 to 15 mg I.V. Nursing considerations include observing for respiratory

depression, changes in level of consciousness, and decreased urine output; and evaluating drug effectiveness.

2. Streptokinase (Streptase)--this thrombolytic activates plasminogen, which dissolves blood clots. Dose range: 250,000 IU, I.V., over 30 minutes. Nursing considerations include monitoring the client for any bleeding; maintaining the infused extremity in a straight position to avoid bleeding at I.V. site; avoiding I.M. injections; observing for allergic reactions; and avoiding unnecessary client handling to prevent bruising.

3. Nitroglycerin (Nitrostat)--this nitrate decreases afterload and increases blood flow through the coronary arteries, thereby decreasing chest pain from angina. Nursing considerations include teaching the client to avoid using alcohol, to use patch regularly as prescribed, and to always have a supply of tablets on hand. Advise the client to take pills at the first sign of an angina attack by placing the tablet under the tongue until all the tablet is absorbed. Teach the client to go to the emergency department if pain persists after taking three tablets spaced 5 minutes apart.

4. Lidocaine (Xylocaine)--this ventricular antiarrhythmic decreases depolarization, automaticity, and excitability in cardiac tissues to abolish ventricular arrhythmias. Dose range: 50 to 100 mg I.V. push at repeated intervals followed by continuous I.V. infusion. Nursing considerations include placing the client on cardiac monitoring, checking blood pressure frequently, and observing for toxicity in at-risk clients.

Nutrition considerations
1. Low-sodium, low-fat, low-cholesterol diet.
2. Modified caloric intake if weight control is necessary.
3. Teach the client to avoid large meals, to eat regularly, and to not hurry while eating.

GUIDE FOR LOW-FAT EATING

Total fat intake for a low-fat diet should be less than 30% of total calories.

Foods low in fats	Foods high in fats
Egg whites (egg substitutes are excellent), non-shell fish, turkey, skinless chicken, milk (skim or 1%), low-fat or "light" cheeses, whole-grain breads, pastry, rice, low-fat crackers, unsaturated oils, lean cuts of meat	Egg yolks, shellfish, whole milk, butter, cream, including non-dairy creamers, cheeses (cream, cheddar, Swiss, Camembert), doughnuts, muffins, biscuits, pies, cakes, chocolate, palm and coconut oils

Cardiac failure

Overview

Cardiac failure (formerly known as congestive heart failure) is the heart's inability to pump blood adequately to supply tissues with sufficient oxygen and nutrients. Causes include cardiac muscle damage resulting from hypertension, atherosclerosis, cardiac muscle degenerative diseases, pulmonary hypertension, and cardiac valvular disease.

Pathophysiology

In cardiac failure, cardiac muscles' contractile properties are impaired. This impairment decreases cardiac output and renal excretion of fluids. Fluid accumulation increases intravascular volume and accounts for many of the characteristic signs of cardiac failure. In left-sided failure, pulmonary congestion occurs when the left ventricle cannot adequately pump blood coming from the lungs. This increases pulmonary pressures and fluid seepage into the lung tissue. Clinical symptoms of left-sided heart failure are dyspnea, crackles, moist cough, fatigue, anxiety, and orthopnea. In right-sided cardiac failure, the right ventricle cannot empty itself completely of blood, forcing a backup in the systemic circulation. Pitting edema, ascites, anorexia, hepatic congestion, jugular vein distention, and weakness are some of the clinical manifestations of right-sided heart failure.

Key assessments and rationales

1. Assess the client's lungs regularly for crackles.
   Crackles will occur from blood backing up in the pulmonary circulation, causing pulmonary edema and potential hypoxia.
2. Auscultate the heart, listening for an S3 sound.
   The presence of an S3 sound may be an early sign of impending pump failure.
3. Assess for presence of dyspnea, crackles, peripheral edema, and jugular vein distention.
   These are all signs of cardiac failure. The extent of their presence provides baseline data.
4. Assess anxiety level of the client and family.
   Decreased oxygenation, restlessness, and fatigue cause anxiety. The family will need support to reduce their anxiety.

Key interventions and rationales

1. Establish a milieu that will promote physical and mental rest.
   Physical and mental stress make the heart work harder.
2. Give prescribed oxygen.

Oxygen improves tissue oxygenation.
3. Maintain high Fowler's position and apply TED stockings to legs.
   Fowler's helps breathing. TEDs aid in preventing venous congestion, which leads to deep vein thrombosis (DVT) and potential emboli.
4. Administer prescribed diuretics.
   Excess fluids increase cardiac workload. Diuretics reduce volume, thereby improving workload.
5. Monitor I&O, fluid and electrolytes, and daily weights; inspect lower extremities for edema.
   Overhydration can increase cardiac workload. Sodium and potassium deficiencies can result from diuretic therapy.
6. Give ordered cardiac glycosides, such as digoxin.
   Digoxin improves cardiac output by increasing contractility and slowing heart rate.
7. Teach the client home care and management of drug and dietary regimens.
   The client should modify daily activities and follow dietary restrictions to minimize recurrence of symptoms.

Drugs commonly used in this disorder
1. Digoxin (Lanoxin)--this cardiac glycoside strengthens contractions of the myocardium, enhances vagal tone, and suppresses some arrhythmias. Dose range: 0.5 mg loading doses I.V. or PO, then daily oral maintenance doses of 0.125 to 0.25 mg. Nursing considerations include taking apical pulse for a full minute and considering not giving if heart rate becomes less than 60/minute or greater than 120 or is unusually irregular. Monitor routine digoxin levels and potassium levels since hypokalemia can increase the risk of digoxin toxicity. Teach the client how to take his own pulse and the symptoms of toxicity: anorexia, yellow-green halos, palpitations, weakness, and nausea.
2. Furosemide (Lasix)--this loop diuretic reduces sodium and chloride reabsorption to promote fluid loss. Dose range: 40 to 80 mg slowly I.V. for pulmonary edema and 10 to 80 mg PO daily for edema. Nursing considerations include monitoring fluid and electrolytes, especially potassium, weight, blood pressure, and pulse. I.V. Lasix should not be given to clients with significant hypokalemia because of the risk of irritable arrhythmias. Teach the client to rise slowly to avoid dizziness, to avoid alcohol, and to take pill early in day to avoid nighttime voiding.

3. Amrinone lactate (Inocor)--this inotropic vasodilator produces vasodilation through a direct relaxant effect on vascular smooth muscle primarily used with clients unresponsive to cardiac glycosides, diuretics, and vasodilators. Dose range: 0.75 mg/kg I.V. bolus over 2 or 3 minutes followed by a maintenance infusion of 5 to 10 mcg/kg/minute. Nursing considerations include monitoring blood pressure and heart rate throughout the infusion. If blood pressure falls, slow or stop infusion and notify health care provider. Don't administer furosemide and amrinone through the same I.V. line because precipitation occurs.

Nutrition considerations
1. Sodium-restricted diet.

FOODS TO LIMIT ON A LOW-SODIUM DIET

- **Mild sodium restriction--2 or 3 grams sodium per day**
  Table salt, smoked or cured meat and fish such as ham, salted fish, bacon, olives, Kosher meats
- **Moderate sodium restriction--1 gram sodium per day**
  All foods under mild restriction, salt used in cooking, canned meats, chicken, fish, and vegetables, frozen vegetables that have salt added, buttermilk, breads, rolls, crackers, most dried cereals, shellfish, prepared cake mixes
- **Strict sodium restriction--0.5 grams sodium per day**
  All foods listed above, foods made with milk products (i.e., ice cream) green vegetables, store-bought candy, excluding hard candy

Note: There are many low-sodium products on the market that may be substituted for the above.

Hypertension

Overview

Hypertension, known as the silent killer, has been arbitrarily defined as persistent blood pressure above 140/90. The limit for the elderly is 160/90. Hypertension is a major cause of multiple organ damage, especially the heart and kidneys. More than 90% of the clients who develop hypertension have *essential* hypertension, which has no known medical cause. More than half of these clients are unaware of the condition.

A prolonged increase in blood pressure produces an increased morbidity and mortality, especially among the elderly. Hypertension is often associated with diabetes, renal, and vascular diseases. Coronary artery disease and cerebrovascular disease occur more often in clients who are hypertensive than in those who are normotensive.

Pathophysiology

The sympathetic nervous system controls the constriction and relaxation of the blood vessels. Stimulation of this system releases norepinephrine constricting the blood vessels. Emotional factors that stimulate the sympathetic nervous system are fear, anxiety, and chronic stress. As the sympathetic nervous system is stimulated, the adrenal glands are stimulated; they release epinephrine, which causes the kidneys to release renin. This ultimately is converted to angiotensin II, causing vasoconstriction. The kidneys retain sodium and water, resulting in increased intravascular volume. All of these factors enhance a hypertensive state.

Key assessments and rationales

1. Assess the client's blood pressure on three visits on each arm while he is standing, sitting, and lying.
   Blood pressure can rise temporarily when a client is anxious, fearful, or angry. Measurements taken on different occasions and in different positions give a more accurate assessment but can be incorrect if approved techniques are not used.
2. Obtain a complete health history.
   A complete health history reveals any stressors that contribute to hypertension and may demonstrate a familial predisposition.
3. Perform a complete physical assessment.
   This gives baseline data and reveals signs of organ dysfunction.

Key interventions and rationales

1. Teach the client dietary restrictions, weight control, exercise

routines, and lifestyle changes needed to manage the disease. *To achieve the goal of lowering blood pressure, the client must understand the need for self-responsibility in managing what changes must be made in living and understand their impact.*
2. Teach the client about disease and why drugs are prescribed and about safety measures to prevent orthostatic hypotension. *Compliance with drug therapy is difficult; clients may feel well and don't understand long-term consequences of hypertension.*
3. Monitor blood pressure at regular intervals and teach the client how to take his own blood pressure, if appropriate. *Self-monitoring blood pressure helps the client participate in his care. Regular monitoring measures treatment progress.*

Drugs commonly used in this disorder
1. Atenolol (Tenormin)--this sympathetic nervous system beta blocker blocks sympathetic nervous system (SNS) stimuli to the heart, slowing the pulse and lowering blood pressure. Dose range: 50 to 100 mg orally every day. Nursing considerations include teaching the client to monitor blood pressure and pulse, to take at the same time each day, and not to withdraw drug suddenly.
2. Captopril (Capoten)--this angiotensin converting enzyme inhibitor (ACE) blocks the formation of angiotensin II, decreasing water retention, which causes arteriole dilation and lowers blood pressure. Dose range: 25 to 150 mg b.i.d. or t.i.d. Nursing considerations include monitoring pulse and blood pressure, monitoring renal studies, teaching the client to report signs of blood dyscrasia (sore throat, fever, palpitations, edema) and not to discontinue suddenly.

NEUROLOGIC SYSTEM
Increased intracranial pressure

Overview

Increased intracranial pressure (IICP) is a sustained increase in intra-skull pressure of greater than 15 mm Hg. The rigid skull vault holds brain tissue, blood, and cerebral spinal fluid (CSF) in a state of equilibrium under normal conditions. An increase in intracranial pressure (ICP) can occur in the presence of increases in volume of any of these components, such as in infection, hydrocephalus, tumor, cerebral edema, or hemorrhage from trauma or ruptured cerebral aneurysm. IICP is a life-threatening condition because of the potential for cerebral hypoxia.

Pathophysiology

Because of the rigidity of the cranial vault, increases in intracranial pressure related to an increase in any one volume reduces the volume of other cranial contents. CSF is most commonly displaced first, then blood volume, then blood flow caused by compression of the cranial vessels. When the ICP reaches arterial pressure, the brain becomes hypoxic and the client experiences deterioration in levels of consciousness, abnormalities in respirations, pupil changes, increase in systolic blood pressure, widening pulse pressure, bradycardia, and cardiac arrhythmias.

ICP is not uniform throughout the cranium. The brain will shift away from the pressure, causing compromised blood flow and possible brain herniation through the tentorium.

Key assessments and rationales
1. Assess the client's neurological status using Glasgow Coma Scale.
   The level of consciousness and neurological status deteriorate as ICP increases. The client may become restless or confused.
2. Assess the client's vital signs.
   With IICP, the pulse pressure widens, heart rate slows, and respiratory pattern may change. Also, the temperature may elevate.
3. Assess the client for vomiting, headache, pupillary changes, and motor impairment.
   These changes all are signs of increasing ICP.

Key interventions and rationales
1. Maintain head and neck in neutral position.
   This helps promote venous drainage and decreases ICP.
2. Elevate the head of the bed 30 degrees or keep flat, as prescribed.
   Elevation may promote cerebral venous drainage.
3. Avoid clustering nursing care activities.
   Multiple procedures at one time can stimulate the client and increase ICP.
4. Monitor I&O, maintaining fluid limitations if prescribed.
   Restricting fluids and diuretic therapy may decrease ICP but also can lead to dehydration.
5. Prevent infection.
   Clients with invasive ICP catheters are at risk for infection. Strict asepsis with dressing changes is required.

Drugs commonly used in this disorder
1. Dexamethasone (Decadron)--this corticosteroid has an anti-inflammatory effect, decreasing cerebral edema. Dose range: 10 mg I.V., then 4 to 6 mg I.M. q6h. Nursing considerations include monitoring weight, blood pressure, electrolytes, and blood glucose, and tapering dose before discontinuing.
2. Furosemide (Lasix) (see under "Cardiac failure," page 190.)
3. Mannitol (Osmitrol) (see under "Spinal cord injury," page 203.)

Nutrition considerations
1. NPO if unconscious.
2. Blenderized food, if client has difficulty swallowing.

GLASGOW COMA RATING SCALE					
Rating three neurological functions gives an overview of the client's level of responsiveness. The lower the score, the less responsive the client.					
I. Eyes open	Score	II. Motor response	Score	III. Verbal response	Score
Spontaneously	4	Obeys	6	Oriented	5
To speech	3	Localizes pain	5	Confused	4
To pain	2	Withdraws	4	Exchanges are inappropriate	3
No response	1	Abnormal flexion	3	Words are incomprehensible	2
		Extends	2	No response	1
		No response	1		

Cerebral vascular accident (brain attack)
Overview
Cerebral vascular accident (CVA), also called brain attack or stroke, is a loss of cerebral function when blood flow to a part of the brain is interrupted. It is the third highest cause of death in North America. Risk factors include hypertension, atherosclerosis, diabetes, sickle cell disease, and substance abuse.

Pathophysiology
There are three types of CVA: thrombotic, embolic, and hemorrhagic. Cerebral infarction occurs when an area of the brain

loses blood supply because of an arterial occlusion. Thrombi and emboli are the most common causes. The affected area of the brain becomes soft and mushy; swelling occurs, followed by necrosis of cerebral tissue. Marked physical and mental dysfunction occurs depending on the area of the brain affected.

In hemorrhagic stroke caused by aneurysm or hypertension, small cerebral vessels rupture, resulting in bleeding into the surrounding brain tissue. The bleeding displaces brain tissue, compressing it and producing ischemia and cerebral edema. IICP almost always results.

Key assessments and rationales
1. Assess the client's neurological function and vital signs.
   Neurological function and hemodynamic stability can deteriorate rapidly. Emergency nursing interventions may be necessary.
2. Assess the client for motor defects.
   Weakness, paralysis, and dysphagia may occur on the left or right side.
3. Assess the client for elimination disorders.
   Disorders of bladder and bowel elimination are common.
4. Assess the client for sensory-perceptual deficits.
   Losses in vision, hearing, cognition, and perception are possible.
5. Assess the client's ability to communicate.
   Receptive and expressive aphasia are common.

Key interventions and rationales
1. If the client is unconscious, implement care protocols (see table on care of the unconscious client, page 198.).
   A goal for managing care of the unconscious client is modifying the immediate environment until he can adapt to it. Maintaining an open airway, preventing complications of immobility, and performing regular neuro checks are important interventions.
2. Position the client to prevent contractures, using trochanter rolls and other assistive devices, and provide skin care and relieve pressure areas.
   Frequent turning and change of position (at least every 2 hours) help prevent contractures and pressure ulcers.
3. Provide range-of-motion exercises.
   Range-of-motion exercises maintain joint mobility.
4. Approach the client from his unaffected side; place needed supplies on this side.
   Staying on the client's unaffected side and keeping objects on that side compensates for visual deficits.
5. Encourage self-care when feasible.

Helping achieve self-care builds the client's morale and prepares him for return to an independent life.
6. Speak slowly and keep instructions consistent. Use the speech therapist's treatment plan.
   Aphasia limits the client's ability to communicate and understand. Slow speaking and consistent instruction creates a milieu conducive to good communication.
7. Establish a bowel and bladder training program.
   Bowel and bladder retraining may be needed if the client is incontinent.
8. Provide home care teaching to the client and family.
   Home care teaching helps the family prepare the home for a client with physical deficits and a possible long-term recovery process.
9. Reassure the family and prepare them for long recovery period.
   The family is important for an optimum recovery. They may have difficulty accepting the client's dysfunction. Community-based stroke groups are available to help the client and family adjust to changes.

Drugs commonly used in this disorder
1. Warfarin sodium (Coumadin)--this anticoagulant inhibits vitamin K activation of clotting factors. Dose range: 10 to 15 mg PO initially, then 2 to 10 mg daily for maintenance. Nursing considerations include teaching the client the importance of compliance and taking drug at same time each day; warning the client not to take aspirin, teaching him to use an electric razor to avoid skin nicks that could bleed excessively, and telling him to report any excessive or unusual bleeding. Warn him that he will have frequent blood drawings to monitor PT or INR.

Nutrition considerations
1. NPO if unconscious. I.V. fluids only.
2. Soft or blenderized foods if the client is unable to chew effectively. Thickened liquids for swallowing difficulties.
3. Enteral feedings may be ordered if the client is unable to swallow.

CARE OF THE UNCONSCIOUS CLIENT

Nursing goals are to adapt local environment to the client's condition and prevent complications. The quality of care given to an unconscious client can be the difference between life and death because of impaired protection reflexes.

• Maintain a patent airway	• Orient to time and place
• Prevent immobility complications	• Perform hourly neuro checks
• Maintain safety (padded bed rails)	• Use seizure precautions
• Patch eyes if corneal reflex is absent	• Provide frequent skin care
• Prevent urine retention	• Maintain oral hygiene
	• Promote bowel function
	• Support the family

Epilepsy

Overview

Seizures are sudden intense episodes of excessive, uncontrolled abnormal cerebral neuronal activity. Epilepsy is a brain disorder characterized by recurring seizures. Seizures are characterized as partial (where the client has no loss of consciousness but exhibits motor, sensory, autonomic, or cognitive symptoms) or generalized (where the client loses consciousness and has severe tonic and clonic spasms). The majority of cases are "idiopathic" (no known etiology evident during life or on autopsy) but seizure disorders often follows brain trauma, drug toxicity, and some infections. Epilepsy usually occurs before age 20.

Pathophysiology

The action of nerves produces electrochemical energy. This energy is what causes a neurological task to be performed. In some pathological conditions or for unknown reasons, the nerves continue to discharge electrochemical energy after the job the nerve had been called upon to do is finished. The parts of the body controlled by the nerve's function respond erratically because of the unwanted discharges of energy. These erratic movements are seizures. Repeated seizures constitute epilepsy.

Key assessments and rationales

1. Elicit the client's seizure history.
   History of seizures helps identify type of seizures and whether the client has epilepsy.

2. Assess the effects of the seizures on the client's lifestyle.
   Lifestyle limitations help identify what modifications may need to be made in the care plan.
3. Ask the client what factors seem to precipitate seizures.
   Knowing precipitating factors will help develop a teaching plan for the client.
4. Get a description of the seizures from the client or family.
   A description of the seizure will help determine the type of seizure and help set a management plan.

Key interventions and rationales
1. Keep the client safe during a seizure; reorient him and provide rest as needed following seizure.
   Preventing injury is the major goal during a seizure. See table, " Interventions during a seizure," page 201.)
2. Reduce the client's fear of seizures.
   Teaching the client to comply with the treatment program will build confidence in the therapy and lower his fear of having another seizure.
3. Help the client improve his coping skills.
   Coping with the constant fear of having another seizure is stressful.
4. Teach the client about the disease, drug therapy, and vocational rehabilitation programs available.
   Counseling should be available to help the client work through the emotions connected with having epilepsy. Embarrassment and social withdrawal are frequent results of epilepsy.
5. Establish a regular schedule for daily activity and medication routine.
   A regular schedule of activity helps avoid things that precipitate seizures. Avoiding the excesses of exercise, overeating, and drinking, and leading a moderate lifestyle will lower the threshold for seizures. Anticonvulsants should be taken regularly at the same time each day to enhance compliance.

Drugs commonly used in this disorder
1. Phenytoin (Dilantin)--this anticonvulsant stabilizes neuronal activity, reducing the release of electrochemical energy that produces uncontrolled nerve activity. Dose range: A loading dose of 900 mg t.i.d., PO, then 300 mg daily (usually in extended-release tablets). Nursing considerations include teaching the client to maintain good oral hygiene, to see a dentist regularly, and not

to stop taking drug; directing the client to take the drug after meals to help avoid gastric upset; and explaining that the drug may make urine turn pink, red, or red-brown.

2. Diazepam (Valium)--this drug suppresses spread of seizure activity produced by epileptogenic foci. It is used for status epilepticus and severe recurrent seizures. Dose range: 5 to 10 mg I.V. or I.M. initially with repeated doses if needed. Nursing considerations include monitoring for bradycardia, respiratory depression, and drowsiness.

Nutrition considerations
1. Regular diet in moderation.

INTERNATIONAL CLASSIFICATIONS OF SEIZURES

The Commission on Classification and Terminology of the International League Against Epilepsy provides a current classification of seizure types.

Partial seizures
- Simple
- No change in consciousness
- Motor symptoms
- Sensory and autonomic symptoms
- Complex
- Conscious impairment only
- Cognitive symptoms
- Affective symptoms
- Psychomotor and psychosensory symptoms

Generalized seizures
- Tonic-clonic seizures
- Tonic seizures
- Clonic seizures
- Absence seizures
- Myoclonic seizures
- Atonic seizures
- Infantile spasms

INTERVENTIONS DURING SEIZURES

The goal in caring for a client having a generalized seizure is to prevent injury, physical as well as psychological.

During a seizure
- Ease the client to the floor to prevent falling
- Protect his head from banging on floor
- Loosen his clothing to prevent constricting neck
- **Do not** force open his jaws in spasm to insert anything--lip, tongue, and teeth injury can occur
- Do not restrain limbs--spastic contractions can cause injury
- Turn the client to his side to facilitate saliva and mucus drainage

After seizure
- Keep the client on his side to prevent aspiration
- Comfort and reassure the client, who may be confused and lethargic, post-seizure
- Make sure that the client is breathing and reality oriented. Short periods of apnea can occur.

Spinal cord injury

Overview

Spinal cord injury can result from fracturing or dislocating one or more vertebrae or damaging the spinal cord or nerve roots or both.

Pathophysiology

Within moments after injury, microscopic hemorrhages appear in the central gray matter of the cord. These hemorrhages increase in size until the entire gray matter is hemorrhagic and necrotic. Hemorrhage and edema are followed by reduced perfusion and development of ischemic areas. Cord swelling increases the client's dysfunction, which can be life-threatening if the injury is in the cervical region.

Key assessments and rationales

1. Do a complete neurological assessment. (See "Increased intracranial pressure," page 193, for details.)
   A complete neurological assessment detects motor and sensory changes, helping to determine the level of dysfunction.
2. Assess the client for spinal shock.
   Symptoms of spinal shock include bradycardia, hypotension, paralysis, loss of sensation, and dysfunction in elimination and ability to perspire.
2. Perform physical assessment to detect other injuries.

Violent physical trauma places the client at risk for having multiple system injuries.
4. Assess family relationships.
Injury can have a long-term-care consequences. Data about family resources help establish a care plan.

Key interventions and rationales
1. Implement emergency management of spinal cord injury (see table, page 203).
Spinal cord injury is an emergency requiring well-planned interventions to reduce secondary injury.
2. Provide adequate oxygenation.
Injuries at C-8 and above impair breathing effort. Oxygen and ventilatory support help prevent spinal ischemia and neuron death.
3. Provide aggressive pulmonary care.
Coughing and deep breathing help prevent pneumonia.
4. Monitor for autonomic dysreflexia.
This reflex response to sympathetic stimulation can be life-threatening. Symptoms include pounding headache, bradycardia, acute hypertension, flushed skin, and changes in sweating.
5. Intervene quickly if autonomic dysreflexia occurs.
Interventions include elevating the head of the bed to decrease blood pressure, alleviating any causes such as full bladder, foley kinks, full bowel, or skin pressure, and administering drugs to lower blood pressure (Hyperstat) and increase pulse (atropine).
6. Prevent complications of immobility and infection.
Provide passive range of motion, adequate skin care, and nutrients. Use sterile technique to avoid lung and kidney infections.
7. Assist the family with emotional support, counseling, community groups, and any teaching needs.
Spinal injuries require long-term care and cause major family stress.
8. Provide information on management of sexual dysfunction.
Sexual intercourse, fertilization, and childbearing may be possible, depending on the level of injury. A counseling referral is appropriate.
9. Provide care for a client with a halo fixation device.
Halo care includes maintaining immobility, assessing skin and muscle function, providing pin care and teaching the client about acceptable activities and home management.

Drugs commonly used in this disorder
1. Dexamethasone (Decadron)--this drug is used to control cord edema (see "Increased intracranial pressure," page 195)

2. Mannitol (Osmitrol)--this osmotic diuretic decreases intracellular water, reducing brain and cord edema. Dose range: 15% to 25% solution I.V. over 1 hour. Nursing considerations include monitoring I&O, vital signs, and electrolytes.

Nutrition considerations
1. NPO until bowel sounds return.
2. Offer liquids with high acid-ash content, i.e., cranberry juice.
3. Offer a high-fiber, vitamin-rich diet. Avoid foods causing flatus.

EMERGENCY MANAGEMENT
OF SUSPECTED SPINAL CORD INJURY

Any motor vehicle accident, sports injury, or direct head or neck trauma should be treated as a potential cord injury.

- Using a back board, immobilize the spine before transporting the client.
- Use at least four people to slide the client onto the board. Absolutely avoid any twisting motion of the client's body.
- Maintain the client in a neutral, extended position. Do not let him sit up.
- When the client arrives in the emergency department, place him on a turning bed (Stryker) or Foster frame.

Parkinson's disease

Overview
Parkinson's disease is a chronic, degenerative neurological disease that affects the brain's basal ganglia, the area responsible for the control and regulation of motor activity. It is characterized by progressive stiff muscle rigidity, tremors, and a shuffling gait. The disease is most often seen in people over age 60.

Pathophysiology
The etiology of Parkinson's disease is unknown. Atrophy and neuronal loss in the cerebral cortex occurs. Dopamine, an inhibitory neurotransmitter, is depleted in the brain. This dopamine depletion and a corresponding increase in cholinergic activity causes tremors and akinesia. Brain blood flow is reduced, causing dementia.

Key assessments and rationales
1. Take a health history.
   A health history focuses on how the disease has affected the client's daily activities and his ability to function normally.

2. Assess the client for tremors, muscle rigidity, and propulsive gait. *Tremors, especially pill-rolling of the thumb and forefinger, are characteristic of the disorder.*
3. Note the client's ability to change position and maintain balance. *A propulsive gait (festination), bending forward, and taking quick short steps on the toes leads to imbalance and frequent falls.*
4. Assess the client's swallowing ability. *Aspiration pneumonia is a frequent cause of death.*
5. Assess changes in the client's lifestyle caused by symptoms. *Forced lifestyle changes can cause depression and living problems for the family.*
6. Observe the client's relationship with his family. *Stress and anxiety will likely develop in the family because of the marked physical and mental changes that occur with the disease.*

Key interventions and rationales
1. Develop an exercise and walking routine; institute physical therapy. *An exercise program will build muscle strength, decrease muscle rigidity, and improve the client's coordination.*
2. Help the client build ways to increase self-care activities. *Increasing the ability to self-care builds self-esteem and promotes independence.*
3. Monitor nutrition and bowel elimination. Have the client sit upright when eating. *Clients are often unable to chew and swallow easily. Good nutrition must be assured to avoid weight loss and bowel elimination problems. Try to decrease possibility of aspiration. 4. Institute speech therapy. Because the client may have difficulty enunciating or speaking clearly, a speech therapist can teach exercises to improve speech or provide assistive devices to improve communication. Speech therapist can also help with dysphagia.*
5. Provide emotional support and teaching to the family. *Helping the family understand Parkinson's disease, involving them in care planning, and offering information about community support groups and national organizations can help loved ones cope.*
6. Help the client minimize sleep disturbances. *Interventions such as limiting day-time napping, decreasing evening caffeine, alcohol, and nicotine intake, and providing a restful environment may help eliminate common sleep pattern disturbances.*

Drugs commonly used in this disorder
1. Carbidopa-levodopa (Sinemet)--this antiparkinsonian drug

counters the depletion of dopamine in the brain. Dose range: three to six 25/100-mg tablets daily in divided doses. Nursing considerations include teaching the client to take the drug with food; monitoring blood pressure; and adjusting dose according to the client's response.
2. Selegiline hydrochloride (Eldepryl)--this MAOI increases dopamine uptake. Dose range: 10 mg PO daily in two divided doses. Nursing considerations include warning the client about dizziness, especially at start of drug, and teaching him not to eat tyramine-containing foods and to have blood pressure monitored. This drug may cause fatal interactions with opioids.

Nutrition considerations
1. Regular diet in semi-solid form with thick liquids. This food form is easier to swallow for clients with swallowing difficulties.

Alzheimer's disease

Overview

Alzheimer's disease is a common degenerative neurologic form of dementia that causes progressive and irreversible deterioration of cognitive functioning. The cause is unknown but the disease is considered familial. Memory loss usually is the first sign of the disease, followed by deterioration of cognition, intellect, judgment, physical decline, and loss of ADL function.

A tangled mass of non-functioning neurons and neural plaques occur in the cerebral cortex, resulting in cerebral atrophy. Chemical changes occur as a result of decreases in acetylcholine, norepinephrine, serotonin, and somatostatin neurotransmitters. The three stages of Alzheimer's disease progress from memory loss to cognitive impairment, finally increasing dependence for daily living. Life expectancy from time of diagnosis is 7 years.

Key assessments and rationales
1. Assess the client's physical status, paying special attention to coordination, vision, ability to chew and swallow, and continence. *A physical assessment provides baseline information about the client's ability to function in the home environment or need to be hospitalized.*
2. Assess the client's mental status, ability to concentrate, reality orientation, and memory loss (both short- and long-term). *Knowing mental status helps plan interventions that best meet the client's needs.*
3. Ask about the impact of client's behavioral changes on the family.

The client's deteriorating condition may leave the family embarrassed, guilty, or ashamed of his behavior.

4. Establish a base of family's knowledge about long-term consequences of the disease and their ability to care for the client. *The family will need help managing home care. Knowledge of how the disease progresses lets the family plan realistically for the future.*

Key interventions and rationales

1. Arrange for a home visit by the home care nurse every 3 weeks and as necessary. *Frequent home visits let the nurse observe changes that may develop in the client's ability to function. The family can be encouraged to discuss feelings about caring for the client at home.*

2. Establish a daily routine for hygiene care, eating, exercise, and recreation. Provide rest periods between activities. *A daily routine helps the client stay oriented and know what to expect during the day. Rest periods are necessary because clients tire easily.*

3. Always address the client by name and identify yourself when interacting. *Helps keep the client oriented to self and caregivers.*

4. Label furniture and clothes. *Labeling furniture and clothes helps avoid confusion and gives dignity to the client who may not want to reveal memory loss.*

5. Develop a meal plan. *A regular meal schedule will remind the client when to eat. Familiar food cut in pieces creates enjoyment during the meal.*

6. Provide safety guards around the house, especially the bath. *This helps minimize risk of injury because of confusion and disorientation.*

7. Develop a toileting schedule. Pay attention to amount of fluid intake. *A toilet schedule reminds the client to go to the bathroom, reinforces memory, and encourages continence.*

8. Provide emotional support for the family and initiate contacts with community agencies. *Groups like the Alzheimer's Foundation can give the family emotional support and help keep the client out of an institution.*

9. Encourage social interactions with family and friends. *This keeps the client oriented, and family and friends stay connected.*

Drug commonly used in this disorder

1. Tacrine hydrochloride (Cognex)--this is the first medication approved for mild to moderate Alzheimer's disease. Tacrine

blocks the breakdown of ACh, which helps enhance memory and reasoning. Dose range: 10 mg PO q.i.d., then up to 40 mg q.i.d. if tolerated. Nursing considerations include having the client take on an empty stomach; monitoring liver studies; observing for GI bleeding; and titrating the dose to client tolerance. Teaching includes monitoring compliance, not stopping the drug suddenly, and avoiding nicotine products.

Nutrition considerations
1. Well-balanced diet of simple, tasteful foods the client likes. If possible, give the client choice in selecting food.
2. Food should be warm, not hot, and cut in small pieces.
3. Limit fluids during the evening hours to avoid incontinence.
4. Provide adequate fiber.
5. Avoid stimulants (coffee, tea, cola, chocolate).

PROBLEMS AND SOLUTIONS IN CARING FOR CLIENTS WITH ALZHEIMER'S DISEASE

- **Wandering**
  Provide a safe place for wandering.
- **Incontinence**
  Establish a toileting schedule (i.e., q2h).
  Use adult diapers (i.e., Depends) if needed.
- **Self-care deficits**
  Provide the structure/assistance needed.
  Limit choices.
  Lay out clothing in the order to be put on.
  Offer simple, easily handled foods.
- **Social withdrawal**
  Do not plan "surprises."
  Let the client determine who can be around.
  Provide the client with familiar activities, calm surroundings.
- **Confusion/disorientation**
  Label objects in the environment.
  Keep surroundings simple.
  Do not use puns and jokes.
  Color-code possessions.
  Use the client's name and state your name when addressing him.
- **Social inappropriateness**
  Stay close to the client in social situations and provide the direction and structure needed.
- **Emotional lability**
  Maintain a calm demeanor.
  Use a quiet tone of voice.
  Give prescribed medications, if needed.

HOME CARE TIPS
FOR COGNITIVELY IMPAIRED CLIENTS

1. **To prevent falls:**
   - Cover or remove extension cords.
   - Eliminate throw rugs.
   - Correct uneven surfaces.
   - Install handrails on stairs.
   - Install fitted carpet in bathroom.
   - Use a skid-resistant mat in tub or shower.
   - Have bright lighting around stairs or rises.
   - Avoid slick floors.
   - Be sure there are no unnecessary objects on the floor.
   - Have hand rails in shower or tub.
   - Put a gate at the head of flights of stairs.
   - Use floor-level shower rather than tub shower.

2. **To prevent burns:**
   - Lower temperature on water heater.
   - Wrap uninsulated hot water pipes.
   - Put a barrier in front of radiators, pot-belly stoves.

3. **To prevent accidental poisoning:**
   - Put poisonous substances out of reach or in a locked cabinet.
   - Remove any poisonous houseplants.
   - Place small objects such as pins, buttons, or tacks out of reach or securely store them away.

4. **To prevent fires:**
   - Remove knobs from the stove.
   - Ask gas company how to inactivate a gas stove.
   - Place matches out of sight and out of reach.
   - Install special deactivating device on electric stove.

5. **To prevent accidental harm to self or family members:**
   - Lock away firearms and other potential weapons (darts, bow and arrow, scissors, knives).
   - Install safety devises on machinery and power equipment and lock away.
   - Remove and secure keys to automobile.
   - Remove locks from bathroom and bedroom doors.
   - Install locks high on outside doors to prevent wandering away from the home during the night.

RESPIRATORY SYSTEM

Tuberculosis

Overview

Tuberculosis (TB) is an infectious disease caused by the mycobacterium tuberculosis. It had steadily declined as a major illness in the United States with the introduction of antituberculosis drugs. Recently, the disease has begun to increase alarmingly. It is a major world-wide health problem, even though it is considered a preventable disease. Drug use, HIV epidemic, and resistant strains are thought to be the reason for the increase of the disease.

Pathophysiology

The mycobacterium is transmitted by air through talking, coughing, sneezing, and laughing. Droplets remain suspended in air and are inhaled by a person susceptible to the disease. The bacteria become lodged in the alveoli and multiply. An anti-inflammatory response results in many dead bacteria, causing an initial pneumonia. The masses of dead bacteria are enveloped by granular tissue walling off the bacteria (GHON tubercle). The disease becomes dormant until the immune system is compromised or reinfection occurs. The lungs become inflamed and pneumonia develops, leading to the formation of more tubercles.

Key assessments and rationales

1. Do a complete history and physical noting anorexia, night sweats, fever, weight loss, and sputum production.
   These are the classic signs of TB.
2. Assess lungs for consolidation, crackles, fremitus, and dullness.
   This provides additional data to aid in the diagnosis.
3. Assess the client's living conditions and understanding of the disease.
   Cramped, dirty housing accommodations, and association with persons who are actively infected increase the likelihood of contracting TB.
4. Perform a tuberculin skin test.
   The Mantoux Test is a skin test that determines if a person has been infected with TB. The size of the resulting induration indicates active infection.

Key interventions and rationales

1. Assure adherence to drug treatment regimen.
   Newly diagnosed cases of TB in the United States are treated with

three antitubercular drugs--isoniazid (INH), rifampin, and pyrazinamide. Compliance with at least 6 months of initial therapy is essential for treatment and to help prevent development of drug-resistant strains of the tuberculi bacillus (MDR-TB).

2. Teach the client normal hygiene measures to prevent the spread of TB.
Hygienic measures such as using tissues to cough into, covering mouth and nose when coughing and sneezing, and frequent handwashing prevent the spread of TB.

3. Teach the client and family how to perform techniques to remove airway secretions.
Secretions block airway passages and interfere with adequate gas exchange.

4. Develop a plan for ensuring that the client has an adequate diet.
Clients with TB may have limited resources for acquiring good nutrition. Designing meal plans and identifying places where a good meal can be obtained helps ensure good nutrition.

5. Provide directly observed therapy (DOT) for persons in high-risk groups.
With DOT health care providers or a designated person must directly observe the client as he ingests anti-TB medications to ensure adherence to prescribed therapy.

6. Teach the client and family about home care.
Teaching the family about good hygiene and the importance of making sure the client takes the drugs prescribed on time will increase the likelihood of successful treatment.

Drugs commonly used in this disorder

1. Isoniazid (INH)--this antitubercular drug inhibits cell wall synthesis by interfering with lipid and DNA synthesis. INH is used in combination with rifampin and pyrazinamide. Dose range: up to 300 mg/day for 6 months to 2 years. Nursing considerations include teaching the client to take with food and to avoid alcohol; monitoring liver function; and ensuring cooperation with regimen.

Nutrition considerations

1. Small, frequent meals to avoid fatigue in a probably debilitated client.
2. Liquid nutrition supplements (i.e., Isocal) to increase daily intake of calories.

Chronic airflow limitation

Overview

Chronic airflow limitation (CAL), formerly known as chronic obstructive pulmonary disease (COPD), is a collection of disorders; chronic bronchitis, bronchiectasis, emphysema, and asthma. It is irreversible, although its progression can be slowed with prompt intervention. CAL is a disease of genetics and the environment. Cigarette smoking and air pollution are factors that contribute to acquiring the disorder. It is the fourth most common cause of death, preceded only by heart disease, cancer, and stroke.

Pathophysiology

CAL is a disease of airway obstruction. There is a decrease in lung elasticity from chronic infection and inflammation of the respiratory tree, resulting in decreased expiratory flow rate. Bronchial constriction from asthma is caused by hyper-reactivity of the smooth bronchial musculature. In emphysema, the distension of and destruction of alveolar walls becomes irreversible. Chronic bronchitis leads to chronic bronchial inflammation, which narrows the airways and produces a lot of thick, tenacious secretions. Continued airway obstruction results in prolonged expiration and impaired gas exchange.

Key assessments and rationales

1. Assess the client's exposure to risk factors.
   Heredity, smoking, and exposure to pollution contribute to development of chronic airflow limitation.
2. Note respiratory difficulties such as dyspnea, shortness of breath, and characteristic posture.
   Dyspnea, especially on exertion, and leaning forward with arms propped on a table are characteristic findings.
3. Auscultate lung fields for wheezing and hyperresonance.
   Alveolar hyperinflation causes hyperresonance; collapsed airway produces wheezing.
4. Note any cough and whether it is productive.
   This is a common symptom of chronic airflow limitation.
5. Assess what changes have occurred in the client's lifestyle.
   Because of the extreme fatigue caused by fighting to breath, the client may have stopped working, cannot exercise, and has trouble eating and sleeping.
6. Assess for symptoms of right-sided heart failure (cor pulmonale).
   Cor pulmonale can occur in chronic bronchitis. Symptoms include ascites, edema, jugular vein distension, and weight gain.

Key interventions and rationales

1. Explain the danger of smoking to the client and teach him cessation techniques.
   Smoking contributes to further loss of lung function from lung irritation.
2. Teach pursed-lip and abdominal breathing techniques.
   Pursed-lip breathing slows expiration, helping prevent collapse of alveoli. Abdominal breathing increases ventilation while slowing respiratory rate.
3. Perform postural drainage and teach the technique to the family.
   Postural drainage uses gravity to raise secretions so they may be expectorated or suctioned.
4. Provide oxygen therapy as prescribed and monitor arterial blood gases (ABGs) and pulse oximetry.
   Chronic high level carbon dioxide levels may decrease breathing stimulus. Oxygen should be administered at low levels to avoid respiratory suppression. Pulse oximetry and ABGs help monitor for hypercapnia and hypoxemia.
5. Teach the client physical conditioning and breathing exercises.
   Good physical condition enhances stamina, muscle strength, and ventilation.
6. Teach the client how to use inhalers and about other medications.
   Proper use of inhalers is essential. Beta agonists and anticholinergics should be inhaled prior to corticosteroids for maximal effectiveness.
7. Teach the client the symptoms of infection.
   Clients should avoid infectious situations that place them at risk for pneumonia. Fever, increased fatigue, change in sputum, or cough should be reported.

Drugs commonly used in this disorder

1. Albuterol (Proventil)--this bronchodilator works by relaxing bronchial smooth muscle by acting on $beta_2$-adrenergic receptors. Dosage rage for adults and children aged 12 and over varies. For aerosol inhalation, one or two inhalations every 4 to 6 hours; oral tablets, 2 to 4 mg PO t.i.d. Nursing considerations include monitoring for nervousness and tachycardia, and teaching the client to wait at least 2 minutes before repeating aerosol inhalation if more than one inhalation is ordered.
2. Ipratropium bromide (Atrovent)--this inhaled bronchodilator inhibits vagally mediated reflexes by antagonizing acetylcholine.

Dose range for adults: one or two inhalations q.i.d. Additional inhalations may be needed, but total inhalation should not exceed 12 in 24 hours. Nursing considerations include using cautiously in clients with angle-closure glaucoma, and teaching the client that this drug is not effective for treating acute episodes of bronchospasm where rapid response is required.

3. Theophylline (Theo DUR)--this bronchodilator relaxes the smooth muscles of the bronchi. Dose range: 3 mg/kg q8h up to 900 mg per day. Nursing considerations include monitoring the client for restlessness and tachycardia; checking serum theophylline levels; and teaching the client to take with water and to avoid crushing or chewing slow-release products.

4. Prednisone (Deltasone)--this adrenocorticoid decreases inflammation by suppressing the immune response. Dose range: 5 to 60 mg PO daily. Nursing considerations include monitoring for heart failure, hyperglycemia, hypertension, edema, infections, GI ulcerations, hypokalemia, and for clients on long-term therapy, concern for osteoporosis, and muscle weakness. Teach the client not to discontinue the drug suddenly, to take with food, to carry a medic-alert card, and to be aware of long-term cushingoid symptoms.

Nutrition considerations
1. Lots of fluids to liquefy secretions. Teach the client to keep fluids close by as a reminder to drink.
2. Small, frequent meals will avoid fatigue and prevent compromised respirations because of a full stomach.

Lung resection

Overview
Full or partial resection of a lung is a surgical procedure for treating lung cancer, bronchiectasis, or lung abscess. Chest tubes are required because the pleural space has been invaded, interrupting the normal negative pressure in the chest.

Clients undergoing a resection of all or part of the lung usually have compromised breathing. They require intensive preoperative and postoperative nursing care to assure survival.

Pathophysiology
Any invasion of the pleural space causes changes in intrathoracic pressure. Normal ventilation (process of air movement) is based on

the principle of negative pressure. The loss of this negative pressure collapses the lung on the affected side. Air, blood, or other fluids can collect in the pleural space and compromise pulmonary function by restricting lung expansion. Chest tubes and a closed chest drainage system (usually a commercial system, such as Pleur-evac or Thyrocele, is used in preference to a bottle system) remove the air and fluid and let the lung expand.

Key assessments and rationales

1. Do a complete physical assessment, paying attention to smoking history, breathing pattern, position assumed when sleeping, sputum production, and ability to perform ADLs.
   A physical assessment identifies risk factors that need to be considered in the care plan.
2. Assess oxygen saturation with pulse oximetry and note crackles or wheezes on auscultation.
   Baseline information will help direct postoperative care plan.
3. Assess the client's emotional state about his disorder and surgery. Evaluate the family's ability to provide support during home care.
   The client's fear of the surgery, motivation to recover, and the family's ability to provide emotional support during the recovery period need to be addressed.

Key interventions and rationales

1. Preoperatively, teach the client and family what to expect during the postoperative period. Teach coughing and breathing techniques.
   Preoperative teaching will encourage compliance with coughing and breathing exercises postoperatively.
2. Explain that mechanical ventilation may be used postoperatively.
   This reassures the client and relieves his anxiety related to ventilator use.
3. Maintain a closed chest tube drainage system.
   Taped connections prevent inadvertent tube removal or disruption of system.
4. Keep chest drainage tubing straight and free of kinks; maintain patency.
   These could interfere with drainage.
5. Check chest drainage water seal chamber frequently.
   Water level in the water seal chamber should fluctuate with respiratory effort; water in the suction chamber should bubble gently when suction applied.
6. Measure chest drainage every 8 hours.

Bright red drainage indicated hemorrhage. Cloudiness could indicate infection.

7. Encourage deep breathing and coughing; use incentive spriometry (IS) as prescribed.
   These promote lung expansion and secretion drainage.
8. Promote mobility. Change the client's position frequently.
   This aids in promoting comfort, helps breathing, and prevents complications of immobility.
9. Provide pain relief through prescribed patient-controlled analgesia (PCA).
   Severe pain can decrease coping and deep breathing. A PCA pump gives the client control pain management in an expedient fashion.
10. Teach the client arm and shoulder exercises.
    These exercises help maintain normal range of motion.
11. Teach home care to the client and family.
    Clients should be taught breathing techniques; the importance of regular exercise, nutrients, and rest; to avoid respiratory irritants and persons with infections; and to report symptoms of complications.

Drugs commonly used in this disorder
1. Cefoxitin sodium (Mefoxin)--this cephalosporin antibiotic inhibits bacterial cell-wall synthesis. Dose range: 1 to 2 g q8h I.V. Nursing considerations include doing sensitivity test before first dose; monitoring for thrombophlebitis at I.V. site; and observing for diarrhea or allergic rash. Avoid using if the client is sensitive to penicillins because cross-sensitivity can occur.

Nutrition considerations
1. Liquid diet after bowel sounds return.
2. Small, nutritiously balanced meals until full recovery.

MUSCULOSKELETAL SYSTEM
Hip fracture
Overview

Fractures of the hip are one of the most common problems of the elderly. Osteoporosis, weak muscles, generalized frailty, pathologic fractures, and drug effects all are factors that contribute to the high incidence. The goals of fracture management include re-establishing bone union, restoring joint mobility, and returning the client to an ambulatory status. Hip fractures have a high mortality among clients over 70 years of age and may be catastrophic for the client and family. Immediate medical intervention and intensive nursing care are high priorities. Surgical treatment is preferred to restore mobility as quickly as possible. Buck's extension may be used temporarily until surgery can be done.

VIEW THE PROGRAM *"CARE OF CLIENTS IN TRACTION"* BEFORE PROCEEDING. IT IS THE 7TH AND LAST PROGRAM ON THE VIDEO MODULE.

Pathophysiology

Two major types of hip fracture can occur: *intracapsular*, which is a fracture of the femoral neck and *extracapsular,* which is a fracture of the trochanter of the femur (See illustration below).

When a fracture occurs, circulation to the periosteum, bone cortex, bone marrow, and the tissue surrounding the fracture is damaged. Hemorrhage results from rupture of the intermedullary circulation, often leading to hemorrhagic shock (see section on "Shock," page 50). Bone and tissue begin to die from loss of circulation, which causes a severe inflammatory response, resulting in intense pain. Peripheral numbness can occur from severing or pinching of the adjacent nerves. Muscle spasms develop, causing pain and a shortening of the affected limb.

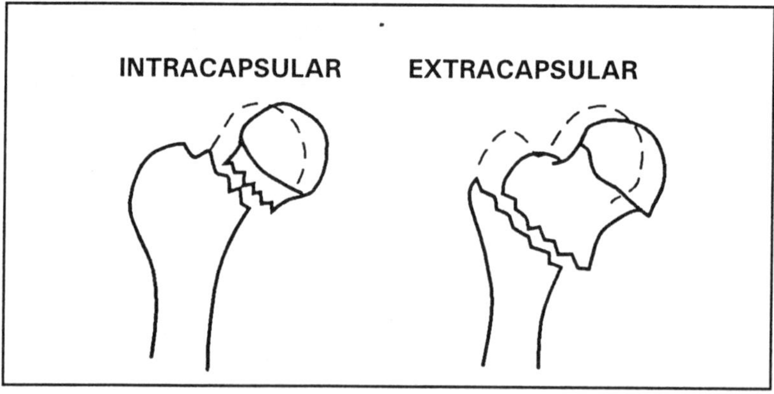

Key assessments and rationales

1. Check the client's vital signs and level of pain.
   Hip fractures can cause serious internal bleeding, leading to shock. Pain level will determine analgesic needs.
2. Assess the client's level of consciousness and mental state.
   Elderly clients may be confused and disoriented and unable to comply with treatment protocols.
3. Check application of skin traction (Buck's extension), if used.
   Buck's extension stabilizes fracture and relieves spasms and pain.
4. Assess the client's hydration and nutrition status.
   Many clients are found a long time after the injury. They may be dehydrated and probably will not have eaten.

Key interventions and rationales

1. Monitor the client's vital signs.
   Blood loss and stress can lead to shock.
2. Note character and amount of drainage. Measure thigh circumference and compare to unaffected limb.
   Excess drainage of bright red blood suggests hemorrhage. Thigh measurement can detect bleeding into tissue, which is not readily observable.
3. Perform regular neurovascular checks.
   Neurovascular checks will alert to complications that could compromise return to normal function.
4. Reposition client q2h. Positions are limited if Buck's extension is in place. Provide skin care at regular intervals.
   Changes in position will help reduce pain and prevent pressure ulcers.
5. Keep the client oriented to environment.
   Keeping the client oriented will promote understanding and compliance with treatment and decrease risk of injury.
6. Ambulate the client to a chair using a walker as soon as possible.
   Early ambulation prevents complications and promotes a quicker return to normal function.
7. Provide pain relief.
   Pain control enhances healing and reduces stress.
8. Promote deep breathing and use of IS.
   Breathing exercises, including IS, prevent complications.
9. Do discharge teaching for return to home or rehab facility.
   Rehabilitation at home may be lengthy and require modification of the home and physical help with ADLs.

Drugs commonly use in this disorder

1. Acetaminophen (Tylenol)--this non-narcotic analgesic blocks pain impulses in the CNS. It is available mixed with narcotics, especially codeine. Dose range: 325 to 650 mg PO q4h, not to exceed 4 g daily. Nursing considerations include teaching the client not to take OTC medicines that may contain Tylenol; and using cautiously in clients who abuse alcohol. Caffeine may enhance effect. Overdose causes hepatic toxicity.

2. Enoxaparin sodium (Levenox)--this low-molecular-weight heparin derivative is used to prevent DVT following hip surgery. Dose: 40 mg subcutaneously (SC) once daily for 7 to 10 days. Initial dose given 12 hours prior to surgery. Nursing considerations include assessing the client for confusion; monitoring platelet count; and instructing the client to watch for signs of bleeding and to notify health care provider immediately.

Nutrition considerations

1. Liquid to regular diet as tolerated.
2. Add supplementary vitamin C and D or serve foods with high vitamin C and D content to clients with suspected osteoporosis.

PERFORMING NEUROVASCULAR CHECKS

Check	Rationale
• Tissue color and temperature	• Indicates circulation status; should be warm and not discolored.
• Nail bed capillary refill	• Normal perfusion, if refill in 2 or 4 seconds.
• Edema and swelling	• Presence may mean venous stasis or tissue injury.
• Range of motion	• Identifies limitations.
• Sensations	• Numbness or tingling indicate nerve pressure.
• Pain	• Means injury, pressure, and/or trauma.
• Peripheral pulses	• Indicate perfusion of limb.
• Bilateral limb tissue	• Provides comparison with healthy tissue on non-injured side.

Rheumatoid arthritis

Overview

Rheumatoid arthritis (RA) is a diffuse connective tissue disease characterized by chronic pervasive inflammation and degeneration of connective tissue. The history of the disease consists of acute flare-ups and remissions. Pain, joint swelling, and hand and feet deformities cause chronic stress and body image disturbances in clients with RA.

Medical treatment involves the aggressive use of NSAIDs and gold compounds early in the disease. Corticosteroids are used later when the inflammation becomes unremitting. Surgery is used to correct marked extremity deformities.

Pathophysiology

An autoimmune reaction occurs in the synovium (the tissue that lines the joint cavities), producing severe inflammation. An enzyme produced by phagocytosis causes edema and a breakdown of cartilage. The attendant loss of mobility results in muscle degeneration and contractility, further exacerbating the problem.

Key assessments and rationales

1. Assess functional limits on mobility of joints. Inspect for bilateral and symmetrical involvement and for deformities.
   Impaired mobility and limb deformity cause stress and limit ability to function.
2. Assess the client's pain level and duration.
   Pain is an integral part of RA. Verbalization leads to identifying factors that increase pain.
3. Determine the client's fatigue level, his rest and activity patterns.
   Fatigue is directly related to the disease activity. Knowing the extent of fatigue helps plan measures to reduce it.
4. Evaluate the client's knowledge of disease.
   The client will need to make lifestyle modifications, and knowing about RA will make these easier.

Key interventions and rationales

1. Promote planned rest and restorative sleep periods.
   Physical and mental rest reduce fatigue. Quality sleep periods help manage constant pain.
2. Maintain optimal joint mobility, with focus on rest in acute exacerbations.
   Good joint position (a position of extension rather than flexion)

helps prevent deformity.
3. Provide comfort measures such as analgesics, heat, cold, and relaxation techniques.
   Comfort measures help the client cope with the chronic pain. Relaxation techniques reduce fatigue.
4. Monitor for drug adverse effects and infection.
   Drug therapy is aggressive and can have adverse effects, which cause anxiety and further stress as well as possible physical complications.
5. Teach the client how to manage self-care; provide occupational/physical therapy referrals as appropriate.
   Adaptive equipment may need to be introduced to maintain the client's independence.
6. Give emotional support; refer the client to the Arthritis Foundation and local support groups.
   Emotional support reduces fear and helps clients cope with RA.

Drugs commonly used in this disorder
1. Acetylsalicylic acid (aspirin)--this nonnarcotic analgesic produces analgesia by blocking prostaglandin synthesis. Dose range for adults, 2.4 to 3.6 g PO daily in divided doses. Nursing considerations include teaching the client to take aspirin with food or milk, and observing for signs of gastrointestinal bleeding.
2. Ibuprofen (Motrin)--this NSAID is an anti-inflammatory and analgesic. Dose range: 200 to 800 mg PO not to exceed 3.2 g a day. Nursing considerations include teaching the client that it will be up to 4 weeks before he will feel the drug's full effect; teaching him the signs of GI toxicity and that he should report any GI bleeding; telling him to take the drug with milk to avoid GI upset and to avoid using with aspirin and alcohol.
3. Aurothioglucose (Solganal)--this gold compound alters immune response and provides an anti-inflammatory effect. Dose range: 10 g I.M. initially, then 50 mg weekly until 1 g given. Nursing considerations include monitoring for bradycardia, renal failure, and toxicity. Teach the client to report rashes and a metallic taste, to avoid sunlight, and that effects won't occur for 3 or 4 months.

Nutrition considerations
1. Weight-reduction diet to reduce pressure on joints, if client is overweight.

Gangrene with limb amputation

Overview

Gangrene is the death of tissue from tissue hypoxia, resulting from arteriosclerosis or other peripheral vascular diseases. It is a common complication of DM and Raynaud's disease. Burns, frostbite, or crushing injuries can also cause gangrene. The untreated condition spreads throughout the affected limb. Gangrene of an extremity from peripheral vascular disease is the most often cause for limb amputation.

Pathophysiology

Poor tissue oxygenation leads to cell death, which results in necrosis. This necrosis is an irreversible state and may be accompanied by invasive bacterial growth in surrounding tissue. The tissue becomes dry, shriveled, and turns brown to deep black. A heavy foul odor is often present from the accumulated pus. The local necrosis produces an inflammatory response in surrounding tissue, leading it to become infected and gangrenous.

Key assessments and rationales

1. Assess the client's general physical health.
   This establishes a baseline of data and indicates the client's ability to endure anesthesia and surgery.
2. Check the neurovascular status of the affected limb, comparing it to the unaffected limb.
   This provides data on the limb's range of motion and its circulatory function, and it indicates tissue perfusion, which will be important in planning postoperative rehabilitation.
3. Check for enlarged lymph nodes, fever, and purulent drainage.
   Systemic infection is likely to be present and antibiotic therapy will have to be started.
4. Evaluate nutritional state.
   Often an elderly client may be poorly nourished. An altered nutritional state will require a vitamin supplement and a high-caloric diet to promote wound healing.
5. Assess the client's mental state and emotional reaction to impending amputation.
   Fear of disfigurement and future immobility will compromise the client's recovery.

Key interventions and rationale

1. Preoperatively, explain the procedure to the client in simple terms, giving him time to express his concerns and fear.

This helps reduce anxiety and provides comfort.

2. Have a healthy amputee visit the client.
   This shows him that people can adjust and provides emotional support from one who has experienced an amputation.
3. Postoperatively, monitor the client's vital signs.
   This permits early detection of complications.
4. Monitor the stump dressing, if any.
   Serosanguinous drainage normally may be present. The initial dressing may be left intact for 24 hours to stabilize the wound. Amputations are either open (the tissue is cut straight across and remains open) or closed (healthy skin is sutured over the amputated wound). If the amputation was open, the client returns to surgery later for closure.
5. Monitor the stump for color, edema, drainage, and signs of infection.
   This gives information about healing and alerts the nurse to the developing complications.
6. Elevate the stump on a pillow and in a neutral position.
   Elevating the stump decreases edema, and a neutral position lessens development of contractures.
7. Make sure that a tourniquet is at the bedside if the client had an open amputation.
   Hemorrhage is always a risk. If it occurs, apply the tourniquet 3 inches above the amputation and notify the surgeon. Immediate ligature of the bleeding vessel is required.
8. Check for evidence of phantom pain.
   Phantom pain, the complaint of pain or feeling in the missing limb, varies in intensity and results from tissue hypoxia and preoperative infection.
9. Ambulate the client on the day of surgery. Use crutches or walker if a leg was amputated.
   Early ambulation prevents complications and starts the client on the road to rehabilitation. If the client is weak and dizzy, help him walk. Teaching good posture helps maintain balance because changes in the center of gravity may have occurred.
10. Perform limb exercises daily; position the client prone intermittently.
    Flexion, extension, abduction, and adduction exercises build strength and help prevent contractures. Prone position prevents flexion contractures, which would later interfere with mobility.
11. Monitor the client for complications such as hemorrhage, infection, and skin breakdown.

These common complications may prolong recovery or endanger the client's life. Poor circulation or a contaminated wound often cause postoperative infection. Poor circulation may require higher amputation to reach healthy tissue that can heal. Good skin care and a limb sock will protect the skin.

12. Teach the client and family home care.

Effective rehabilitation requires involvement of all the client's family. Having a functional prosthesis is one goal of rehabilitation. The family will need to know about referrals to other health workers, i.e. physical therapist, physiatrist, and vocational counselors.

Drugs commonly used in this disorder

1. Ampicillin sodium/sulbactam sodium (Unasyn)--this combination of aminopenicillin/beta-lactamase inhibitor inhibits cell wall synthesis and inactivates beta-lactamase from destroying the ampicillin. Dose range: 1.5 to 3 g I.V. or I.M. q6h. Nursing considerations include checking for allergies to penicillins; not mixing with other I.V. drugs; and watching for diarrhea or hypersensitivity rash. Change I.V. site q48h to prevent vein irritation.

Nutrition considerations

1. Regular balanced diet as tolerated. Add vitamin supplements to diet if client is debilitated or malnourished, especially vitamin C for tissue healing.

HOME-CARE TEACHING FOR AMPUTATION

Achieving independent self-care and a return to normal function requires thorough teaching of the client and family.

- Do regular, daily washing of stump with soap and water; assess for signs of irritation.
- Modify home for the client using walker or crutches.
- Tell the client that if the stump skin is irritated, he should not wear the prosthesis but should call the home care nurse.
- Teach the client how to apply stump sock smoothly when arising for the day.
- Elevate limb q4h for 20 minutes; extend limb to prevent flexion contractures.
- Use tepid bath water to prevent burning.

INTEGUMENTARY SYSTEM

Burns

Overview

About 70,000 people are hospitalized each year because of burn injuries. The most common place this injury occurs is in the home. Factors associated with burn injury are age, smoking, intoxication, occupation, and the presence of physical or mental disease.

Burns are caused by heat, electricity, radiation, or chemicals. The very young and the very old have the highest mortality following burns because of their bodies' inability to cope with the massive multisystem damage that can occur in severe burns. Burns are categorized as minor, moderate, or major injuries.

Pathophysiology

Minor and moderate uncomplicated burn injuries damage the epidermis and some dermis. Pain and redness occur, but the skin maintains its ability to withstand bacterial invasion and loss of water.

Major partial- or full-thickness burns destroy the entire epidermis, dermis, and subcutaneous tissue. Muscle and bone also may be damaged or destroyed. Multisystem pathology occurs in major full-thickness burns, hypovolemic shock being the most life-threatening. Intravascular fluids leak into the interstitial spaces (fluid shift), quickly leading to hypovolemic shock. Hyponatremia occurs because of fluid shift. Hyperkalemia results from cellular destruction. Hypermetabolism occurs in direct proportion to the area burned. All pathophysiology is in direct proportion to the extent of body area involved. Pain is present in minor, superficial moderate, and partial-thickness burns. There is no pain in full-thickness burns.

Key assessments and rationales

1. Check the client's airway for patency and character of respirations.
   If the client inhaled smoke, airway obstruction is a risk. Inhalation of smoke, heat, and chemical gases can burn the respiratory tree.
2. Assess the client's vital signs hourly.
   Hypovolemic shock is a high risk for burn clients, particularly if a large body surface has been burned. Vital sign changes are an early indicator of impending shock. (See review of "Shock," page 50.)
3. Assess type of burn and body surface area (BSA) burned using the

"Rule of Nines." (See figure, page 227.)
The burn depth and extent of the area of the body burned will determine the medical and nursing interventions. If the burn area is scattered, use palm method to determine BSA injured. The size of the client's palm is approximately 1%.
4. Perform a complete physical assessment.
A head-to-toe assessment will reveal the presence of other illnesses or injuries. The neurological assessment establishes level of conscious, amount of pain, and the client's anxiety.
5. Check the client's urine output and specific gravity.
Severe burns can cause renal shutdown from hypovolemic shock when fluid shifts occur. Urine output indicates circulatory system status. Specimens should also be checked for myoglobin and hemoglobinuria.

Key interventions and rationales
1. Institute emergency burn management (see table, page 226).
Priority is to stop burning process and support vital functions.
2. Monitor the client's respiratory status, including ABGs and oxygen saturation.
Inhalation injuries can require intubation and ventilation. Provide oxygen and encourage coughing and deep breathing.
3. Monitor the client's fluid and electrolyte status.
Fluid replacement is essential. Physiologic shifts in fluids and electrolytes need careful monitoring and replacement as indicated.
4. Maintain the client's body temperature.
Hypothermia can occur from loss of skin and fluids. Maintain body temperature at 99.6° to 101°F.
5. Provide pain relief.
Burns can cause excruciating pain. Using PCA pumps, guided imagery, relaxation techniques, and ample narcotics are indicated.
6. Provide gastric decompression via nasogastric (NG) tube and maintain adequate nutritional support.
To prevent and manage gastric dilation and ileus, use parental nutrition until the GI system is functional, then enteral feeding until the client can meet nutritional needs PO. Tissue catabolism and a hypermetabolic state are present. Accurate supplementation of caloric needs is essential.
7. Provide adequate wound care.
Deep burn wounds may require hydrotherapy, debridement, and/or surgical management. Aseptic technique is required. Report any sign of infection immediately. Meticulous graft and donor site care will help prevent further disfigurement and/or

immobility.
8. Use proper positioning and encourage ambulation and exercise. *These help to prevent contractures from forming.*
9. Teach the client and family about home care needs. *Rehabilitation can be long term, requiring physical therapy, home modifications, and psychological counseling and support. Referrals to burn support groups may be helpful. Reconstructive and cosmetic surgeries may be required.*

Drugs commonly used in this disorder
1. Silver sulfadiazine--this broad-spectrum sulfonamide antibiotic decreases bacterial folic acid synthesis. Applied topically in 1/16-inch thickness to burn wounds daily or b.i.d. Nursing considerations include using sterile technique and using an analgesic prior to burn care as needed. Monitor for hypersensitivity and agranulocytosis.

Nutrition considerations
1. Nutritional support begins when the client is stabilized.
2. Maintain nutrition support to meet the hypermetabolic state that occurs post-burn (high carbohydrate, high protein).
3. Intake as high as 5,000 calories per day may be needed.

EMERGENCY BURN MANAGEMENT	
These actions should be given priority in on-the-scene management of a burn-injured client.	
Action	**Rationale**
1. Extinguish flames: cut off electrical source.	This protects the emergency crew from injury and stops the burning process.
2. Cool the burn.	Using cool water on the burn area and any adhered clothing stops further burning.
3. Remove any restrictive clothes.	This prevents constriction from edema that will develop quickly.
4. Irrigate chemical burn.	This stops the burning process by diluting chemical.
5. Cover the burn area.	This helps prevent contamination and infection. It decreases pain by blocking air flow over the burn area.

RULES OF NINE

Estimating total body surface area burned is crucial in planning and determining treatment outcomes. First-degree burns are excluded from the estimate.

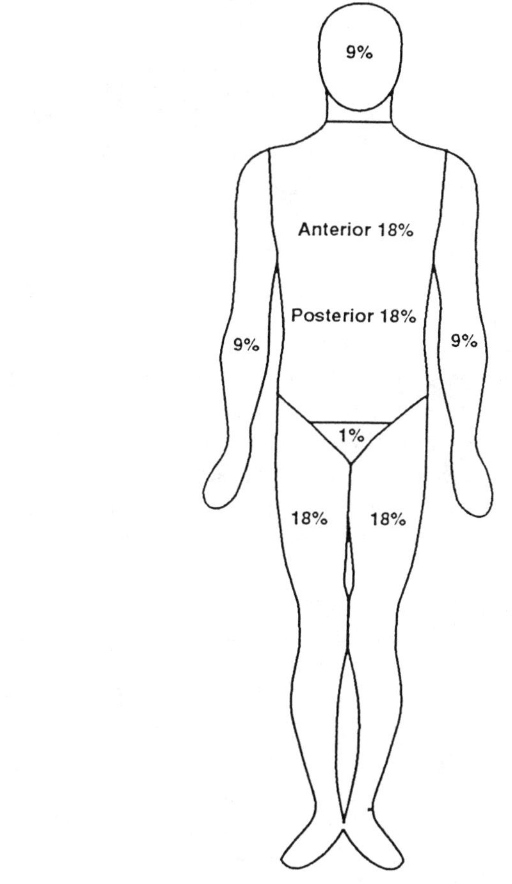

ENDOCRINE SYSTEM

Type 2 diabetes mellitus

Overview

Diabetes mellitus (DM) is a constellation of disorders characterized by glucose intolerance. It is a chronic alteration in the production or use of insulin and is characterized by blood glucose levels consistently elevated above the normal range of 80 to 120 mg/dl.

The majority of people diagnosed with diabetes have Type 2 (non-insulin dependent diabetes). Type 2 DM occurs mainly in clients over age 30 who are overweight and physically inactive. Treatment of type 2 DM usually begins with weight control, exercise, and diet. Antidiabetic drugs are introduced if blood glucose levels remain above normal. In some cases, insulin is required to successfully manage Type 2 diabetes.

Pathophysiology

In Type 2 DM, the pancreas' insulin secretion is impaired and tissue sensitivity to insulin is decreased or resistant. Normally, insulin binds to special receptors on the cell surface, letting it enter the cell. Because of unknown factors, insulin fails to bind to cell receptors and builds up in the blood. Beta cell changes in the pancreas are non-specific in Type 2 DM.

Key assessments and rationales

1. Perform a complete history and physical examination.
   This will establish a baseline and give information about any limitations in the client's ability to learn and comply with treatment plan.
2. Assess the client for polydipsia, polyphagia, polyuria, and weight loss. Assess skin dryness and turgor.
   These are the classic signs of DM.
3. Check the client's vision by asking him to read a newspaper; check his coordination.
   Defects in ability to read or hand-eye coordination will affect the client's ability to comply with the treatment plan.
4. Assess literacy, family, and social support systems.
   The client's daily living schedule will change. Strong family, social, and financial resources will help him comply with treatment.
5. Evaluate the client's emotional state and coping skills.
   This will elicit any fears the client has about diabetes and the coping skills he used to handle past difficulties.

Key interventions and rationales

1. Teach the client about the interaction of diet management, exercise, and medication.
   Type 2 DM can be controlled successfully if the client knows the importance of controlling calories, having a regular exercise routine, and taking antidiabetic medication as ordered.

2. Inspect the client's feet at each visit and teach good foot care.
   Clients with diabetes are prone to peripheral vascular compromise, often evidenced first in foot ulcers. Feet must be washed daily and covered with clean socks. Teach the client not to walk barefoot.

3. Provide emotional support to the client and family.
   Both the client and family may suffer from increased anxiety because of the complexity of activities that need to be learned. Giving positive reinforcement when an activity is performed well builds esteem.

4. Teach basic diabetes survival skills such as recognition of hypoglycemia, diet management, daily hygiene, self-blood-glucose monitoring.
   Successful diabetes management requires the client's complete cooperation. The better he knows how to manage the many details, the better he will be able to comply with them.

5. Monitor the client for complications of diabetes.
   Cardiovascular disease, renal disease, peripheral vascular disease, infections, and retinopathy are long-term complications. A yearly eye exam is recommended along with routine medical care.

6. Continually evaluate the client's ability to comply with the treatment plan.
   Compliance may decrease as motor, visual, hearing, and other abilities decline with normal aging. Care plans should be modified to the client's current abilities.

Drugs commonly used in this disorder

1. Tolbutamide (Orinase)--this sulfonylurea promotes insulin release from the pancreas and enhances tissue sensitivity. Dose range: 500 to 2,000 mg daily in divided doses. Nursing considerations include teaching the client to take drug on schedule, to carry hard candy at all times in case of a hypoglycemic reaction, to avoid large amounts of alcohol, and not to take OTC drugs without his health care provider's permission.

2. Glucophage (Metformin)--this biguanide decreases hepatic glucose production and improves insulin sensitivity. Dose range: 500 to 2,500 mg daily. Nursing considerations include monitoring blood

glucose; teaching client to take the drug with water, to avoid alcohol, to discontinue the drug and call his health care provider if unexplained hyperventilation, myalgia, or malaise occur, and to avoid other drugs unless approved by his health care provider.

Nutrition considerations

1. Calorie-controlled diet to lower and maintain weight at desired level. Teach the client the importance of adhering to diet and exercise to help control diabetes. Arrange for dietary consultation if the client has difficulty complying with meal plan.

HOW TO HANDLE SICK PERIODS

Clients with diabetes will develop a URI or the "flu" just like everyone else. Here is what to teach them when they get ill.

1. Take antidiabetic medications, as ordered.
2. Test blood glucose level three or four times a day using blood-glucose monitor. If above 300 mg/dl, report it to health care provider.
3. If vomiting, take fluids to prevent dehydration and supply calories. Regular cola, orange juice, broth, and sports drinks are good.
4. If unable to eat regular meal plan, eat soft foods like gelatin, custard, or soups.
5. If vomiting and diarrhea last more than 2 days, report it to health care provider.

Cushing's syndrome

Overview

Cushing's syndrome results from a chronic, excessive level of circulating cortisol. The cause may be a tumor of the pituitary or adrenal glands. Long-term administration of cortisone also may cause the disorder. It is more common in women than men, usually occurring between 30 and 50 years old.

The excess circulating cortisol causes weight gain, a characteristic "moon face" and "buffalo hump." About half of clients with Cushing's syndrome have some change in mental status, ranging from simple depression to severe psychiatric symptoms. Because infection is a high risk, more than half of the clients die within 5 years after diagnosis.

Pathophysiology

Primary Cushing's syndrome results from a benign or malignant adrenal tumor that increases cortisol production. High cortisol levels cause changes in fat, protein, and glucose metabolism. Changes in metabolism account for fatty deposits, muscle wasting, skin changes, elevated glucose, osteoporosis, hypokalemia, hypertension, emotional, and endocrine changes.

Key assessments and rationale

1. Assess the client's level of physical activity and ability to carry out ADLs.
   Weakness is a common symptom from the muscle wasting that occurs.
2. Carefully check skin for breaks, infection, and bruising.
   The protein wasting causes thin skin, which is at high risk for infection because of elevated glucose levels.
3. Evaluate mental status, looking for signs of depression and concern about body image changes.
   The marked changes in facial appearance and increased hair growth and weight can lead to depression, irritability, and withdrawal.
4. Determine the family's response to illness.
   The client's physical and mental changes affect the entire family. They need to express feelings and develop coping skills.

Key interventions and rationales

1. Monitor the client for fluid volume excess.
   Accurate measurements of I&O, daily weight, and blood pressure will help prevent fluid volume increase.
2. Provide a protective environment from falls and injury.
   With Cushing's disease, there is a risk of injury from weakened muscles in combination with osteoporosis and fatigue. A safe environment must be provided at all times. Rest periods will help conserve energy and prevent possible injury.
3. Prevent opportunistic infections.
   Elevated cortisol levels impair the immune response and delay wound healing. Clients should have a private room and be protected from sources of infection through aseptic technique and teaching.
4. Provide emotional support to the client and family.
   The disease is debilitating, and body image changes may occur. Offering time to verbalize feelings and ask questions may allay some concerns. Referrals to mental health providers may be necessary.

Drugs commonly used in this disorder
1. Aminoglutethimide (Cytadren)--this drug may be ordered to suppress adrenal function until medical interventions can be instituted. Treatment should begin and continue in a hospital until dosage is stabilized. Dose range: 250 mg PO, q.i.d. at 6-hour intervals. Nursing considerations include teaching the client not to stop drug abruptly; watching for drowsiness and dizziness; and monitoring for orthostatic hypotension.

Nutrition considerations
1. Diet high in protein, calcium, and vitamin D helps reduce effects of muscle wasting and osteoporosis.
2. High-protein diet helps maintain skin integrity.

Hyperthyroidism

Overview
Hyperthyroidism is a disease of excessive secretion of thyroid hormones. It is one of the most commonly seen endocrine disorders, second only to DM.

Graves disease, a multisystem autoimmune disorder, is the most common cause of hyperthyroidism. It occurs most commonly in women under age 40. The cause is unknown but may be related to emotional stress, thyroiditis, or a possible hereditary link.

Pathophysiology
In Graves disease, long-acting thyroid stimulators stimulate the thyroid gland, which increases thyroid hormone. This hyperthyroid state produces the characteristic symptoms of exopthalamos, goiter, fatigue, amenorrhea, tachycardia, restlessness, weight loss, hypertension, and excessive sweating.

Key assessments and rationales
1. Assess the client for exophthalmos, heat intolerance, sweating, rapid pulse and respiration, and emotional state.
   These are the classic signs of hyperthyroidism caused by excess thyroid hormone circulating in the body.
2. Obtain a history of when exaggerated symptoms first occurred.
   This helps pinpoint the precipitating cause of the disease and gives information about the client's current nutritional and emotional status.
3. Assess the client's stress history and ability to cope with increased metabolism.
   Stress is a contributing factor to the disorder. The high level of metabolism exhibited in hyperthyroidism will require strong coping skills.

Key interventions and rationales
1. Monitor for signs of thyroid storm. (See table, page 234..)
   Thyroid storm (thyrotoxic crisis) is severe hyperthyroidism manifested by high fever, extreme rapid pulse, hypertension, and marked mental changes, including delirium.
2. Maintain a quiet, peaceful, and cool environment.
   The client is hyperexcitable, so loud noises, music, or talking can overstimulate him. The high metabolic rate makes him feel unusually warm. A cool room and cool baths will provide relief.
3. Provide emotional support and enhance self-esteem.
   The client will have many frightening feelings. Changes in appearance can make him withdraw from social contact. A calm, understanding approach and careful explanation of all treatments assures both the client and family.
4. Teach the client eye care protection measures.
   Exophthalmus is a common sequela of hyperthyroidism. Eyedrops and eye patches may be prescribed. Teach the client how to instill drops and to use a patch to protect the cornea.
5. Support the client during radioactive iodine (^{131}I) therapy.
   ^{131}I destroys thyroid tissue. Clients are anxious when they hear they are taking radioactive drugs. Because they are sent home after the radioactive drug is given and the incidence of hypothyroidism is very high, teach both the client and family the signs of hypothyroidism. Teach the client that his saliva will be radioactive for about a day and to avoid kissing.

Drugs commonly use in this disorder
1. Propylthiouracil [PTU] (Propyl-Thyracil)--this thyroid hormone antagonist blocks the formation of thyroid hormone. Dose range: 100 mg PO t.i.d. Nursing considerations include teaching the client to report any skin rash, fever, sore mouth, and not to take OTC medicines that contain iodine.
2. Propranolol (Inderal)--this beta blocker blocks catecholamine synthesis and is used to treat cardiac symptoms of hyperthyroidism. It also produces a calming effect in very excited clients. Dose range: 10 to 20 mg PO t.i.d. Nursing considerations include monitoring for bradycardia and hypotension. Teach client not to discontinue drug abruptly and to take the drug with meals to enhance absorption.

Nutrition considerations
1. Small, well-balanced meals served several times a day help satisfy increased appetite.
2. Reduce or eliminate stimulant foods like coffee and cola drinks.
3. Provide nutrition supplements to maintain weight and nutrition.

MANAGING THYROID STORM

Thyroid storm or thyrotoxic crisis is a life-threatening condition brought on by stress, infection, pregnancy, or manipulation of the thyroid gland. It requires immediate intervention.

Signs
1. Profound tachycardia (over 130 bpm)
2. Hyperpyrexia (over 100° F)
3. Weight loss, diarrhea, chest pain, dyspnea, psychological behavior changes

Treatment
1. Reduce heart rate and body temperature to prevent cardiovascular failure. Use hypothermia blanket and give Tylenol (salicylates are contraindicated--they worsen the hyperthyroidism).
2. Give the client oxygen to meet increased metabolism and assure tissue oxygenation.
3. Administer I.V. fluids containing dextrose to replace lost glycogen.
4. Give propylthiouracil to block the formation of thyroid hormone.
5. Treat the client as critically ill until acute phase is over.

Hypothyroidism

Overview

Hypothyroidism results from a decreased amount of circulating thyroid hormones (TH). The disease affects all body systems, producing decreased metabolism, cold intolerance, lethargy, slowed mental processes, and cardiovascular and pulmonary changes. Hypothyroid states in adults are sometimes called myxedema. Myxedema refers to nonpitting edema in the connective tissues throughout the body, causing facial puffiness and tongue enlargement.

Pathophysiology

Hypothyroidism may be caused by congenital defects, loss of functional thyroid tissue with aging, or thyroiditis, or it may develop after treatment of hyperthyroidism with radiation or surgery. The thyroid gland enlarges in a compensatory attempt to produce more hormones. This enlargement is called a simple goiter.

Key assessments and rationales

1. Assess for goiter, dyspnea, edema, cold intolerance, weight gain, constipation, dry skin, and muscle stiffness.
   These are common signs of hypothyroidism.
2. Monitor for changes in vital signs.

TH deficits can result in bradycardia and hypotension. Respirations can become slow and shallow, risking hypoxemia and atelectasis. Temperature may decrease and clients feel cold. Warm clothing or blankets are indicated.

Key interventions and rationales

1. Establish an activity/rest routine for the client based on his energy level.
   This will encourage and permit the client to participate in self-care activities while ensuring adequate rest periods.
2. Encourage adequate fluids and activity.
   Sufficient fluids and exercise are necessary to prevent constipation and improve muscle tone.
3. Provide measures to maintain skin integrity.
   Hypothyroidism causes dry edematous skin at risk for breakdown. Positioning, turning, bathing, cleaning, and using alcohol-free lotions on the skin may be helpful.
4. Provide teaching for life-long hypothyroidism management.
   Clients need information on self-care, compliance with medications, laboratory tests, activities, and symptoms to report to their health care provider.

Drugs commonly used in this disorder

1. Levothyroxine sodium (Synthroid)--this synthetic thyroid hormone stimulates body metabolism. Dose range: 75 to 125 mcg daily, PO as a maintenance dose. Nursing considerations include monitoring blood pressure and pulse during initiation of drug therapy; teaching the client to report chest pain, dyspnea, sweating, or palpitations to his health care provider; and teaching him the importance of complying with medication schedule and routine to maintain a constant level of the hormone. Drug is a life-long replacement therapy.

Nutrition considerations

1. A high-fiber, high-water-content diet to decrease potential for constipation.
2. Teach the client to increase fluid intake daily to promote softer stools.
3. Teach the client to avoid foods containing iodine, i.e.,soybeans, tofu, turnips.

REPRODUCTIVE SYSTEM
Cancer of the cervix

Overview

Cancer of the cervix remains a common disease, but the death rate has decreased because of effective screening with the Pap test. Although the exact cause is unknown, risk factors include multiple sex partners, multiple pregnancies, early sexual experiences, human papilloma virus infections, genital herpes, and cigarette smoking.

Cervical cancers are classified by stages. Stage I is cancer in situ or confined to the cervix. Stage II is cancer involving the vagina. Stage III is cancer spread to the pelvic walls. Stage IV is cancer spread outside of the reproductive tract. Cervical cancer is diagnosed through a Pap smear. Treatments include radiation, colposcopy, laser surgery, and/or hysterectomy.

Pathophysiology

Cervical tissue changes are progressive. Normal tissue is squamous epithelium. Premalignant lesions occur many years before cancerous cells develop. Because of the risk factors, normal squamous cells progressively develop dysplasia, going from mild to severe. Constantly changing female hormone levels affect cellular changes. Cervical tissue changes gradually invade surrounding tissue and, if left untreated, metastasize through the lymphatic system.

THE PAPANICOLAOU SMEAR

Description: Performed to detect cervical cancer, secretions from the cervical opening (OS) are applied to a glass slide, "fixed," and examined microscopically.

Nursing considerations:
1. Teach the client not to douche before test.
2. Assess if the client is menstruating because blood interferes with test interpretation.
3. Teach the client about positive and negative test results. Most women incorrectly think a positive Pap smear means they have cancer.

Key assessments and rationales
1. Perform a complete health history and physical assessment.
   This will elicit symptoms of cervical pathology as well as establish a baseline for future comparison.

2. Assess the client's anxiety about the cancer diagnosis and knowledge base about treatment outcomes.
   Hearing the cancer diagnosis provokes intense anxiety. The client may not have heard all the treatment choices or the prognosis from the health care provider.

Key interventions and rationales
1. Do preoperative teaching if surgery is the treatment plan.
   Clients may be fearful of disfigurement and possible body image changes.
2. Explain surgical procedures and postoperative routines to expect.
   Clients need information on their procedure, be it cryosurgery, colposcopy, or hysterectomy (abdominal, laparoscopic, or vaginal). Information will help lessen anxiety. Give the client and his loved ones time to express their concerns about cancer and the treatments prescribed.
3. Provide discharge and home teaching.
   Teaching should be tailored to the specific client needs. Information should be provided on activities, infection prevention, changes in menstruation, possible need for replacement hormones, sexual intercourse, symptoms to report, and possible follow-up chemotherapy or radiation.

Drugs commonly used in this disorder
Client may receive chemotherapy or radiation. (See "Chemotherapy" in Chapter 3 for nursing care.)

Nutrition considerations
   1. Postoperatively, liquid to regular diet as tolerated.

GASTROINTESTINAL SYSTEM
Peptic ulcer
Overview
Peptic ulcers, also known as gastric, duodenal, or esophageal ulcers, are crater-like breaks in the mucosal wall of the stomach, duodenum, or pylorus. The erosion of tissue may extend to the muscle layers and into the peritoneum. Often caused by the bacteria *H. pylori*, the disorder is commonly found in men over age 40. Excessive smoking of tobacco products, heavy alcohol use, and long-term use of NSAIDs contribute heavily to predisposition for peptic ulcer.

Pathophysiology
The mucosal wall erosion is caused by an increased concentration of

an acid-pepsin enzyme, decreasing the mucosal wall's ability to withstand the action of hydrochloric acid. The compromised gastric mucosal barrier lets hydrochloric acid penetrate the mucosa, digesting the gastric tissue. *H. pylori*, alcohol, NSAIDs, and other irritants contribute to the weakening of the gastric-mucosal barrier.

Key assessments and rationales

1. Assess history of the client's pain.
   Pain, its origin and description, is an important diagnostic tool. Clients will describe it as burning and intense in the abdomen. It usually occurs several hours after eating and is relieved by taking an antacid or eating food.
2. Have the client describe eating habits and typical diet.
   Foods that are gastric stimulants (i.e., spicy foods) tend to aggravate peptic ulcer disease.
3. Assess the client's smoking, drinking, and lifestyle habits.
   A high-tension lifestyle coupled with smoking and alcohol consumption are risk factors.
4. Do a complete physical assessment. Guaiac stool test may reveal occult blood.
   Palpation of the abdomen may reveal upper gastric tenderness. Blood studies may reveal anemia from ulcer bleeding.
5. Assess for presence of *H. pylori* bacteria.
   This organism has been identified as the major cause of peptic ulcer disease.

Key interventions and rationales

1. Teach the client relaxation techniques.
   This will help the client manage stress and quit smoking.
2. Teach the client about medications prescribed and the importance of medication schedule and what adverse effects may occur.
   When clients become symptom free, they may stop taking the drug, which leads to incomplete healing and reoccurrence of symptoms.
3. Monitor the client for hemorrhage.
   Dizziness and nausea may be symptoms of bleeding. Stool should be tested for occult blood.
4. Do preoperative teaching, if surgery is planned.
   Full or partial gastrectomy is done for intractable disease. The client needs to be able to express concerns and know what to expect from procedure and after returning home.

Drugs commonly used in this disorder

1. Cimetidine (Tagamet)--this H_2 histamine antagonist reduces gastric acid secretion. Dose range: 800 mg PO at bedtime.

Nursing considerations include teaching the client not to take with antacids, which inhibit cimetidine absorption, and to avoid smoking cigarettes, which will increase secretion of stomach acid.

2. Tetracycline hydrochloride (Achromycin)--this bacteriostatic inhibits protein synthesis in gram-negative and gram-positive organisms. Nursing considerations include teaching the client to not to take with milk, food, or antacids and to avoid direct sunlight because of photosensitivity.

3. Omeprazole (Prilosec)--this benzimidazole inhibits the activity of gastric acid. Dose range: 20 to 60 mg daily PO in delayed-release capsules. Nursing considerations include teaching the client to take drug as prescribed, swallowing capsules whole. Monitor hydration state to prevent dehydration.

Nutrition considerations
1. Avoid very hot or very cold foods, which increase acid secretion.
2. Do not drink coffee (including decaffeinated coffee) or cola drinks containing caffeine or use meat extracts, which stimulate gastric acid production.

Colon cancer

Overview
Cancer of the large intestine is the second leading cause of cancer deaths in Western countries. The likelihood of occurrence increases in the fifth decade. Although the exact cause is unknown, risk factors include rectal polyps, family history, ulcerative colitis, Crohn's disease, immunodeficiency disease, and a diet high in fat and calories and low in calcium and fiber. The survival rate is improved through early detection with regular physical exams, sigmoidoscopy, and colonoscopy. Bowel resection is the common intervention for colon cancer.

Pathophysiology
Almost all cancers of the large bowel are adenocarcinomas that develop from adenomatous polyps. Tumors usually grow undetected through direct extension into the bowel walls and neighboring tissues, including the stomach, duodenum, small intestine, pancreas, spleen, urinary tract, abdominal wall, and liver.

Key assessments and rationales
1. Assess the client for changes in bowel habits and passage of bloody stool.
   These common signs of colon cancer are the most frequent reasons clients seek care.

2. Assess the client's knowledge about the disorder and outcome.
   Clients are anxious and fearful of dying. Knowing concerns helps plan care.
3. When surgery is confirmed, do preoperative teaching/preparation.
   Show the client how to do bowel prep, use IS,, and leg exercises. Explaining procedure and postoperative routines help lessen anxiety and build confidence.
4. Make sure that all pre-admission lab work is done.
   Clients will be admitted the day of surgery. Lab work not done or on the client's chart will delay surgery.

Key interventions and rationales
1. Provide routine postoperative care.
   This includes turning q2h, using IS, monitoring I&O; taking vital signs; having the client do ankle exercises; and checking the wound for drainage and bleeding. These measures promote recovery and prevent complications.
2. Monitor for passage of flatus and bowel sounds.
   These indicate return of peristalsis and are signs for removal of the NG tube inserted in the operating room.
3. Discharge teach about dressing changes, if any, exercise and rest routine, and symptoms to report to the health care provider or home care nurse.
   The client will be discharged after a brief hospital stay. Knowing what to do at home relieves client and family anxiety, maintains recovery program, and alerts to possible complications.
4. Emphasize follow-up care instructions.
   Because the client is discharged quickly, all follow-up visits must be kept as scheduled to assure uneventful recovery and avoidance of complications.

Drugs commonly used in this disorder
1. Polyethylene glycol-electrolyte solution (GOLYTELY)--this laxative, acting as an osmotic, is used in bowel preparation for bowel examination and surgery. Dose range: 240 ml PO until 4 liters have been taken. Nursing considerations include teaching the client not to mix with flavored drinks such as orange juice or Kool-Aid, to use regular tap water to reconstitute powder, and to take no food for 4 hours before taking drug.
2. Neomycin sulfate (Mycifradin)--this aminoglycoside inhibits protein synthesis of bacteria. Dose range for bowel prep: 1 g PO q1h for 4 hours. Nursing considerations include teaching the client to take fluids while taking the drug, to eat a low-residue diet before starting medication, and to maintain adequate fluid intake.

Nutrition considerations
1. Low-residue diet, preoperatively.
2. NPO until NG tube removed. Then clear liquids to regular diet, as tolerated.

Cirrhosis

Overview
Hepatic cirrhosis is a chronic liver disease caused primarily by alcoholism but also related to chemical exposure, drug abuse, hepatitis, and malnutrition. The symptoms of the disease are a result of the liver's inability to produce clotting factors and albumin, to regulate glucose metabolism, to detoxify substances, and to regulate blood volume. Hepatic dysfunction can lead to encephalopathy, ascites, and esophageal varices.

Pathophysiology
Liver cell dysfunction is the first sign of tissue damage. Cells become inflamed with fatty infiltrates. This blocks the secretion of liver enzymes, which then begin to build up in the blood. The swollen liver cells block normal function of the hepatic (portal) circulation, causing hypertension in the portal system. The reduced ability to process wastes, regulate hormone balance, and aid in the digestion of foods causes multisystem imbalances to occur. In chronic situations, the liver becomes a shriveled fibrotic mass.

Key assessments and rationales
1. Assess the client's general health and physical state.
   Clients may appear severely malnourished and debilitated, manifesting a fever, cognitive disturbances, jaundice, and an enlarged abdomen from ascites. Initial assessment establishes baseline data that will be important in evaluating treatment success.
2. Assess the client for vomiting of blood and blood in the stool.
   Hematemesis and bloody stool may indicate esophageal varices, GI bleeding, and possible coagulation defects.
3. Assess the client's abdominal girth and weight.
   This indicates presences of ascites, which can be painful and disturb other abdominal organs' function.

Key interventions and rationales
1. Maintain fluid intake and adequate diet.
   Fluid intake will prevent skin drying and constipation but must be carefully controlled if the client has ascites. Malnutrition and possible emaciation need to be corrected.

2. Monitor the client's vital signs frequently; assess him for restlessness.
   Changes in vital signs and restlessness are the first indication of possible complications, particularly esophageal and GI bleeding.
3. Weigh the client daily and measure his abdominal girth; assess for dependent edema.
   This provides data about success in reducing edema and ascites.
4. Administer prescribed vasopressin and vitamin K.
   Pitressin reduces portal hypertension and controls water reabsorption. Vitamin K helps reduce likelihood of bleeding.
5. Monitor the client for possible hepatic encephalopathy.
   This is a central nervous system after-effect of cirrhosis. An early sign is a "flapping tremor" called asterixis. Confusion, anxiety, and irritability are other signs.
6. Keep head-of-bed elevated 45 to 60 degrees.
   This helps breathing, which may be compromised from ascites.
7. Teach the client and family home care procedures.
   The client will need much rest, balanced with careful exercise to avoid exhaustion. Visitors should be limited, and environment kept clean to prevent infection. Prescribed diet must be followed because of liver's inability to metabolize foods properly.
8. Assist the client and family with referral information.
   Clients who have alcoholic cirrhosis need referrals to alcohol rehabilitation programs such as Alcoholics Anonymous. Emotional support will be needed to help clients feeling guilty or in denial.

Drugs commonly used in this disorder
1. Vitamin K_1 (AquaMEPHYTON)--this vitamin promotes the formation of prothrombin, aiding in blood coagulation. Dose range: 2.5 to 10 mg, PO, I.M., or SC. Nursing considerations include monitoring for bronchospasm, anaphylaxis, and pro time.
2. Lactulose (Cephulac)--this laxative is used to prevent and treat portal-systemic encelphalopathy, including hepatic precoma and coma in clients with severe hepatic disease. It decreases blood ammonia, probably as a result of bacterial degradation. Dose range: Initially, 20 to 30 g (30 to 45 ml) PO t.i.d. until two or three soft stools are produced daily. Nursing considerations include monitoring serum sodium for possible hypernatremia.

Nutrition considerations
1. Soft-low roughage, modified protein (70 to 100 g daily) diet.
2. Increase carbohydrates to assure 2,000 to 3,000 calories of food intake each day.
3. Fluid and sodium restriction as prescribed.

GENITOURINARY SYSTEM
Renal calculi

Overview
Urinary tract stones (urolithiasis) can occur anywhere in the urinary tract. They can vary in size from barely perceptible to the size of a tennis ball. Calculi occur in men slightly more than women and are first seen when the client reaches the third decade of life. Factors that influence calculi development include infection, urinary stasis, dehydration, hypercalcemia, malignancy, and parathyroid disease.

Pathophysiology
Urinary calculi contain calcium, uric acid, phosphates, magnesium, and oxalates. Stones develop from the formation of crystals (nidus) in the presence of calcium oxalate, calcium phosphatase, or struvite. The crystals get trapped in the urinary tract and slowly attract more crystals and grow into stones. Urine pH affects the development of different types of stones. Alkaline urine tends to increase the chance of calcium stones developing. Ingestion of high-purine foods, like fish and poultry, contribute to acid urine, which produces struvite stones containing magnesium, ammonium, and phosphate.

Key assessments and rationales
1. Obtain a complete health history and perform a physical assessment.
   This will elicit any conditions that contribute to stone formation and identify the client's physical problems.
2. Have the client describe his pain, its intensity and location.
   Acute pain in the renal area, called renal colic, is a characteristic sign of renal stones.
3. Obtain blood and urine specimens.
   Urine pH, uric acid, and calcium levels are helpful in identifying the type of stone. An elevated WBC count may indicate infection.
4. Assess diet history.
   The type of diet a client eats may contribute to stone formation.

Key interventions and rationales
1. Force fluids, up to 4 liters a day.
   This will dilute urine, reduce the concentration of crystals, and help flush out the urinary tract.
2. Administer anticholinergics, as prescribed.
   Anticholinergics relax the bladder and ureteral muscles, aiding in the passing of small calculi.
3. Strain all urine.
   This will reveal if the calculi has passed through the urinary tract. Straining will collect any calculi for laboratory analysis.
4. Provide pain relief.

Renal colic has been described as the most intense kind of pain. Strong analgesics may be required.

5. Teach the client proper diet to eat according to type of stone that has formed and how to force fluids.
Diet is the most important therapy to prevent calculi development. Increasing knowledge will enhance compliance.

Drugs commonly used in this disorder

1. Methantheline bromide (Banthine)--this anticholinergic blocks acetylcholine, relaxing muscles. Dose range: 50 to 100 mg q6h PO. Nursing considerations include teaching the client to take the drug a half hour before meals, to be careful when driving and engaging in potentially dangerous activities, and to report any skin rash, dizziness, or blurred vision.

Nutrition considerations

1. Forced fluids and a high-acid or high-alkaline diet depending on type of stone found. See table for food choices.

FOOD GUIDE FOR CLIENTS WITH RENAL CALCULI

Diet therapy has an important role in keeping clients free of urinary stones. Teaching what foods to eat and avoid is an important nursing function.

Urine-acidifying foods: Fish, veal, lamb, chicken, beef, pork, prunes, cranberries

Urine-alkalinizing foods: Milk and its products, navy beans, citrus fruit, dried apricots and figs, beet greens, and chives

Foods to avoid if stones contain calcium or oxalate: Cheeses (except cottage), milk products, organ meats, whole grain breads, rice (brown), cereals (except Corn Flakes and Rice Krispies), spinach, beets, tomatoes, all berry fruits, nuts and peanut butter, chocolate

---

Acute renal failure

Overview

Acute renal failure occurs when the body is unable to remove metabolic wastes or carry out the regulatory functions of the kidneys. It is a multisystem disease disrupting metabolic and endocrine functions. Risk factors include hypoperfusion, nephrotoxins, trauma, infection, hemorrhage, heart failure, liver disease, surgery, and lower tract obstruction. Treatment may involve dialysis.

Pathophysiology

Acute renal failure is the sudden cessation of kidney function. Oliguria (urine output less than 400 ml daily) is the most common manifestation of renal failure. Initially, there is a decrease in perfusion of the kidneys with oxygenated blood. This leads to damage of the basic kidney unit, the nephron. Treatment must begin immediately to avoid a complete irreversible shutdown of the kidneys.

Key assessments and rationales

1. Assess electrolytes and I&O.
   This gives data on kidney function and the state of body's electrolytes.
2. Assess the client for the cause of renal failure.
   Shock from cardiovascular disease or hypovolemia and prolonged infection are some possible causes for the failure.
3. Analyze laboratory studies, noting BUN and creatinine levels.
   BUN rises steadily and creatinine rises as the kidney glomeruli become damaged.
4. Evaluate the client's and family's knowledge of the disorder.
   This is a life-threatening condition. The client needs emotional support and the family will need to know the realistic outcomes.

Key interventions and rationales

1. Assist with correcting the underlying disease process that caused the failure.
   Acute renal failure cannot be reversed without correcting the cause, such as infections.
2. Monitor I&O.
   This helps identify whether intake is greater than output and notes the pattern of urinary output, if any. Provide only enough fluid intake to equal the urinary output.
3. Monitor acid/base and electrolyte imbalances.
   Clients are prone to developing acidosis and hyperkalemia, both of which are life-threatening.
4. Weigh the client daily and maintain him on prescribed low-protein diet.
   Glucose utilization and catabolism of protein is impaired. Weight changes are an excellent monitor for detecting fluid retention.
5. Provide frequent mouth and skin care.
   Urea and other waste products are excreted through the mucous membrane and skin. Cool water baths and oral hygiene reduce irritation and pruritus associated with uremic frost.
6. Administer prescribed stool softeners.

High urea levels in the blood and accumulation of organic acids will irritate the colon. Stool softeners will provide comfort.

7. Prepare the client for dialysis.
   Dialysis is the recommended treatment to prevent complications of renal failure. Emotional support and careful explanation of the procedure will relieve anxiety and promote compliance.

Drugs commonly used in this disorder

1. Sodium polystyrene sulfonate (Kayexalate)--this potassium-removing resin exchanges sodium ions with potassium ions in the intestine. It removes excess potassium from the body. Dose range: 15 g one to four times a day. Nursing considerations include monitoring serum potassium levels carefully to prevent hypokalemia; observing the client for sodium overload; and monitoring him for constipation and possible fecal impaction.
2. Sodium docusate (Colace)--this stool softener promotes increased liquid in stool. Dose range: 50 to 300 mg daily. Nursing considerations include giving liquid form in milk or juice to disguise bad taste. Discontinue drug if stomach cramps occur.

Nutrition considerations

1. Low-protein diet to prevent accumulation of waste products. Caloric makeup is with carbohydrates.
2. Low-sodium and low-potassium diet. Restrict fluid intake.

FOODS HIGH AND LOW IN PROTEIN

In a low-protein diet, protein is limited to 1 g/kg of body weight. Protein ingested should be of high biologic value.

High-protein foods: Eggs, milk, cheese, meat, fish, poultry
Low- or zero-protein foods: Butter and sugar ball, Controlyte, Hycal, Polycase, low-protein pasta, cereals, breads

---

NURSING CONSIDERATIONS
FOR CLIENTS HAVING DIALYSIS

Peritoneal dialysis
- Initially, have the client void to prevent bladder puncture.
- Warm dialysate to prevent abdominal pain.
- Place the client in semi-Fowler's and explain procedure.
- Monitor the client's vital signs q15 min to alert to shock or excessive fluid loss.
- Reassure the client and keep him informed during this lengthy process.
- Monitor the client for nausea, respiratory distress, and pain from pressure of fluid in abdomen.

Hemodialysis
- Teach the client about procedure, its purpose, adverse effects, diet restrictions, and care of shunt site.
- Give the client and family time to ask questions and clarify responsibilities.
- Routinely assess the client for signs of depression, which is common because of the severe alterations in lifestyle.
- Monitor the client's compliance with diet and medication therapy.
- Monitor for complications such as infection, shunt obstruction, pruritus, and hypotension.

COMMUNICABLE DISEASES

Viral hepatitis

Overview

Hepatitis is a worldwide public health concern. Five different types of viral hepatitis have been identified; more are suspected. The disease is highly communicable and can strike people of any age. The older the client when infected, the greater the morbidity and mortality. Because so many people infected with a hepatitis virus are asymptomatic, there is a great chance of infection among health care workers. Vaccines against type A and type B hepatitis have afforded significant protection for health care personnel. Prevention of the spread of the infection is an important nursing priority.

Pathophysiology

Each type of hepatitis (see table, page 250) has its own etiology, transmission mode, and disease course. The liver pathology is the same.

The virus, regardless of type, invades, reproduces, and damages only the liver cells. Inflammation, hepatic cell necrosis, accumulation of necrotic wastes, and ultimate cell destruction produce structural changes in liver cells, disrupting bilirubin excretion. The loss of excretory function leads to a buildup of bilirubin in the body resulting in the jaundice seen in many clients with hepatitis.

Hepatic cellular regeneration occurs simultaneously with the hepatic necrosis. Complete regeneration takes 3 or 4 months, which explains the long recovery period.

Key assessments and rationales

1. Assess the client's lifestyle history.
   Hepatitis spreads by use of shared I.V. needles, sexual intercourse, contaminated blood products, and food.
2. Do a physical assessment and take a health history.
   This will identify classic signs of weight loss, mild fever, hypotension, anorexia, nausea and vomiting, joint pain, itching, and presence of jaundice.
3. Assess the client for malaise and fatigue.
   These signs are common and care will have to be planned accordingly.
4. Establish the client's knowledge about the disease and prevention measures.
   Teach preventive care measures to avoid infection with another type of hepatitis and to prevent transmitting the disease to another person.

Key interventions and rationales

1. Make sure that the client can perform ADLs.
   Most clients will get home care. Because of the extreme fatigue and generalized malaise, the client may not desire or be physically able to do daily hygiene measures.
2. Teach the client and caregivers the principles of enteric and universal precautions for this type of disease.

The client can be highly infectious during the acute phase. Take enteric precautions for hepatitis A and E; universal precautions for hepatitis B, C, D, or all.

3. Provide adequate nutrition and fluid intake.
   Anorexia is a typical symptom. Foods of high biologic value the client likes should be presented. Fluids should be forced.
4. Assist with range-of-motion exercises and teach the client and caregivers a rest/exercise schedule tailored to the client's fatigue level.
   The recuperative period is as long as 6 months. The client will need to maintain muscle mass and strength.
5. Teach about the disease and prevention measures.
   Ignorance of how the disease is acquired is common. Knowledge helps prevent reinfection with another type and spread to others. Clients in high-risk categories should be advised to be vaccinated for types A and B.

Drugs commonly used in this disorder
1. Interferon alfa-2b (Intron A)--this biologic modifier seems to interfere with viral replication. It has had good results in chronic cases of hepatitis B and is being used for hepatitis C. Dose range: 5 million unit SC daily for 16 to 24 weeks. Nursing considerations include making sure that the client is not allergic to phenol, a drug preservative; teaching the client to take the drug at bedtime to avoid associated drowsiness, to keep the drug cold, and to report for all follow-up visits.

Nutrition considerations
1. High-protein, high-caloric meals during anorexic phase to maintain nutrition level. Small, frequent meals composed of foods the client likes are better tolerated.

COMPARING TYPES OF HEPATITIS					
	Type A	**Type B**	**Type C**	**Type D**	**Type E**
Route of transmission	Fecal/oral; water-born, contaminated shellfish	Blood or blood products; sexual intercourse; contaminated needles	Transfusion of blood and blood products	Same as C; I.V. drug use	Fecal/oral
Average incubation period	30 days	70 to 80 days	50 days	35 days	42 days
Symptoms	May be absent; headache and other flulike symptoms. Extreme malaise and fatigue, dark urine, jaundice, tender upper right quadrant.	Same as A; rash, easy bruising, joint pain	Same as B	Same as B	Same as A; pregnancy increases severity.
Treatment	Bed rest, high-caloric/ protein diet, forced fluids Enteric precautions	Same as A: interferon may help if disease course is prolonged Universal precautions	Same as B Universal precautions	Same as B Universal precautions	Same as B Enteric precautions
Outcomes	Good; low mortality (<1%), no carrier state	Major cause of cirrhosis; mortality as high as 10%; carrier or chronic hepatitis state	Chronic carrier state. High risk of liver cancer	Same as B	Same as A; prolonged in pregnancy.

Source: *American Nursing Review NCLEX RN* (4th Edition). © 1999 Springhouse Corporation

Acquired immunodeficiency syndrome

Overview

Acquired immunodeficiency syndrome (AIDS) is an incurable collection of illnesses resulting from infection with the human immunodeficiency virus (HIV). More than 10 million people are infected worldwide. The disease is most prevalent among those who engage in high-risk behaviors, such as unprotected homosexual sex, I.V. drug addiction, heterosexual relations with HIV-positive partners. Others at risk are recipients of blood and blood products contaminated with HIV and children born to mothers with the HIV infection.

Transmission is by exchanging body fluids in sexual relations, direct exposure to the virus through contaminated needles, receipt of contaminated blood products--although now rare--and in utero from mother to child.

Pathophysiology

HIV is a retrovirus that binds to certain lymphocytes (CD4+ cells) and injects its genetic material into the cell. The virus begins to replicate and destroys the cell, releasing more viruses into the circulation, where they are transported throughout the body. Virus production is dependent on the health state of the infected person. Healthy people may not develop symptoms of AIDS for 10 years after initial infection. The continued destruction of CD4+ cells compromises the immune system, and the body becomes susceptible to a wide range of opportunistic infections that normally have no effect.

Key assessments and rationales

1. Assess results of HIV test and the client's understanding of its meaning.
   Clients who are seropositive react in profound psychological ways. Panic, depression, and a sense of utter hopelessness prevail.
2. Assess the client for fatigue, chronic respiratory infections, diarrhea, muscle weakness, emaciation, changes in behavior, and skin diseases.
   These are all signs that the HIV-positive client has developed AIDS.
3. Identify the client's support systems.
   The effects of AIDS on the client's physical, emotional, financial,

and social status is overwhelming. Extreme malnutrition and organ failure tax the client's coping abilities.

Key interventions and rationales

1. Provide skin care.
   Skin cancers (Kaposi's sarcoma) and generalized emaciation lead to skin breakdown. Frequent changes of position, meticulous attention to avoiding pressure abrasions, and the use of lotions and non-abrasive soaps help keep skin intact and free of infection.
2. Monitor the client's bowel habits.
   Diarrhea depletes fluids and electrolytes as well as irritating the perianal skin. Measure quantity and volume of liquid stool to determine replacement fluids. Teach the client to avoid bowel-irritating foods like fruits, spicy foods, carbonated beverages, and vegetables.
3. Provide respiratory therapy for ineffective airway clearance.
   Pulmonary conditions like pneumocystic disease are common and compromise the ability to remove pulmonary secretions. Keep the client in a high Fowler's position and encourage frequent coughing and deep breathing to improve airway clearance.
4. Monitor the client for anger, depression, ataxia, eye changes, hallucinations, tremors, and cognitive slowing.
   These manifestations are common. As the disease progresses, the neurological changes can disrupt the family and caregivers.
5. Provide an attitude of acceptance and understanding.
   Clients with AIDS may feel guilty, ashamed, and alone. Often they are isolated by family, friends, and companions. Fostering an opportunity to express feelings and emotions helps clients understand they are not alone.
6. Teach the client about drug therapy regimen and help him get financial assistance.
   The client must take drugs on time around the clock. There is considerable expense with purchasing drugs, so he may need to know how to get financial aid.
7. Encourage the client to engage only in safe-sex practices.
   This prevents transmission of the virus to sex partners.
8. Prevent contamination to health care workers (see table, page 253).
   Nurses always should practice universal precautions when caring for a clients with communicable diseases.

Drugs commonly use in this disorder
1. Zidovudine (Retrovir)--this antiretroviral agent prevents the replication of the HIV. Dose range: 200 mg PO q4h around the clock. Nursing considerations include teaching the client the importance of not missing any dose of the drug, to avoid taking any other drugs not prescribed by the health care provider (they may interfere with Retrovir action), to avoid pregnancy, and to adhere strictly to follow-up visits.
2. Saquinavir (Invirase)--this protease inhibitor binds to the virus protein, preventing it from reproducing. Dose range: 600 mg t.i.d. after a meal *and* in combination with zidovudine. Nursing considerations include teaching the client to take the drug within 2 hours after a meal, to avoid taking any other drugs not prescribed by the health care provider, to avoid breast-feeding while taking this drug, and to report any adverse reactions immediately to nurse or health care provider.

Nutrition considerations
1. High-protein, high-carbohydrate diet composed of foods the client likes. Offer small, frequent meals after providing oral hygiene. Viscous lidocaine may help clients with mouth sores to swallow easier.
2. Offer commercial nutrition supplements like TEN and Advera, a supplement specially formulated for AIDS clients.

UNIVERSAL PRECAUTIONS TO PREVENT HIV SPREAD	
1. Handle all sharp items (needles, scalpels, blades) with care.	6. Be especially cautious if pregnant.
2. Dispose syringes, needles blades in puncture-resistant containers.	7. Flush blood and body fluids down the toilet when working in the home.
3. Wear gloves, gowns, and masks to prevent exposure to blood and body fluids.	8. Wrap contaminated linen, towels, and bandages before discarding in an approved solid waste disposal area.
4. Wash hands and other body parts contaminated with body fluids.	9. Clean body fluid spills with soap and water, household detergent, or 1:10 bleach solutions. Wear gloves.
5. Use mouth pieces and resuscitation bags for CPR.	

Adapted from U.S. Department of Health and Human Services: *Universal precautions for prevention of transmission of HIV and other blood-borne pathogens.*

ONCOLOGY

Breast cancer

Overview

Cancer of the female breast is one of the most common types of cancer in women. Even with improved education about breast self-examination (BSE), the incidence continues to rise. The mortality is unchanged in spite of advances in therapy.

There is no known specific cause of breast cancer, but risk factors have been identified. These include a personal or family history of the disease, having a first child after age 30, starting menses early (before age 12), history of benign breast disease, late menopause, obesity, and exposure to radiation.

Pathophysiology

There are several type of breast tumors, each of which will affect the treatment and prognosis. Generally, tumors don't develop quickly. From the beginning of a genetic alteration in breast cells to the development of a palpable tumor may take several years. The malignant tissue grows and metastasizes throughout the breast tissue ducts and breast lobules. Left untreated, the metastasis spreads to the lymph nodes that drain the breast, then the muscle of the chest wall. Treatment is by surgery, radiation, chemotherapy, or a combination of the three.

Key assessments and rationales

1. Assess the client's response to diagnosis and available coping mechanisms.
   A diagnosis of cancer provokes fear, anxiety about disfigurement and spouse's reaction, and loss of femininity. Knowing how the client has coped with crisis in the past will help develop intervention strategies.
2. Establish the client's knowledge base about the disease, treatment options, and potential outcomes.
   Ignorance is still widespread about how breast cancer is treated. Many clients do not know that there are non-surgical alternatives as well as surgical techniques that do not disfigure.
3. Assess for any discomfort.
   The client may be having pain or muscle discomfort from the disease.

Key interventions and rationales

1. Teach the client about treatment options.
   The client may be experiencing severe anxiety and will need time, patience, and sensitivity in getting information about available treatment.
2. Explain biopsy procedure and how she will participate in treatment decisions.
   The client needs to know what to expect at biopsy and how she will be active in deciding the therapy.
3. If the client is having a mastectomy, teach post-mastectomy exercises like rope climbing and wall walking.
   These prevent postoperative immobility and actively involve the client in the care program.
4. Encourage discussion of fears and perceived loss of femininity.
   Fears and concerns can be discussed during routine postoperative care. Having a person who has had a mastectomy visit the client can provide emotional support and serve as a role model.
5. Teach the client about chemotherapy, radiation therapy, and adverse effects, if she is scheduled for this treatment.
   Knowledge relieves anxiety. The client will need to know limitations on lifestyle and adverse effects of treatment.

Drugs commonly used in this disorder

1. Methotrexate (Folex PFS)--this cell-cycle-specific antineoplastic destroys cancer cells. Dose range: 15 to 20 mg PO daily for 5 days. May be given I.M. Nursing considerations include teaching the client about adverse effects, to report bruising or bleeding, fever, or chills, to manage alopecia, and to use a sunblock when outside.
2. Cyclophosphamide (Cytoxan)--this non-specific alkylating agent interferes with cancer cell growth. Dose range: 40 to 50 mg/kg I.V. over several days. Nursing considerations include teaching the client about adverse effects (especially hair loss, which is reversible), to protect herself from trauma that may cause bleeding, to avoid pregnancy while taking the drug, and to drink 3 liters of fluid daily to avoid hemorrhagic cystitis.

Nutrition considerations

1. Liquid to regular diet postop.
2. Small, frequent soft-food diet during chemotherapy because of mouth sores.

Critical Thinking Exercise

Medical/Surgical Nursing

Facts and objectives
1. The NCLEX-RN tests your ability to make sound clinical judgments.
2. Developing critical thinking skills is the foundation for being able to make good clinical judgments.
3. This exercise will help you evaluate how well you think critically.
4. As you work through this exercise, you will learn how the continuous flow of questions that evolve as you think the case through will lead you to reach solid conclusions about the client problem and the *best* nursing behaviors.

Instructions
Respond to the following questions by writing down your best thoughts, ideas and "answers" in the space provided. Do this for all of the questions, then turn the page to see what you should have considered in response to each question.

Naturally, to learn to think critically, don't look for hints or answers before completing all questions...don't cheat yourself! How you answer the critical questions will depend on how well you perfect your thinking skills.

Overview

A 52-year-old client had an uneventful total abdominal hysterectomy and bilateral salpingo-oophorectomy earlier this morning. The pathology report confirms stage II endometrial cancer with minimal lymph node involvement. She was widowed 6 months ago, has no children, works as a first-grade teacher and has a close relationship with her sister, niece, and two nephews who live nearby. Postoperatively she has a Hemovac attached to an abdominal drain, is receiving an I.V. of D_5LR at 125 ml/hour and has morphine available by PCA pump. You are assigned as her nurse on a general surgical floor.

1. What are your priority assessments?

2. How would you best evaluate this client's pain?

3. What are the goals for this client in the first 24 hours?

4. Describe interventions to prevent common postoperative complications for this client.

5. What are her likely psychosocial nursing diagnoses?

6. What are the discharge teaching needs for this client?

THE FOLLOWING ARE INTERVENTIONS AND NURSING BEHAVIORS YOU SHOULD HAVE CONSIDERED IN ANSWERING THE PREVIOUS QUESTIONS.

1. **What are your priority assessments?**
   - *Incisional dressing, Hemovac drainage, vital signs, level of consciousness, respiratory rate (related to morphine), peripheral circulation, urinary output.*

2. **How would you best evaluate this client's pain?**
   - *Ask the client to assess and rate the intensity of her pain on a rating scale. Assess location, duration, quality, effects of activity, and PCA therapy. Assess for behavioral changes (i.e., grimacing, guarding). Assess for physiological changes (changes in vital signs).*

3. **What are the goals for this client in the first 24 hours?**
   - *Experience minimal pain and discomfort.*
   - *Experience no complications (DVT, bleeding, wound infections, urinary problems, etc.)*
   - *Experience minimal anxiety (able to verbalize issues related to loss of fertility, body image, impact of cancer diagnosis).*
   - *Verbalize knowledge of self-care (turning, leg exercises, deep breathing, ambulation, I&O).*

4. **Describe interventions to prevent common postoperative complications for this client.**
   - *Leg exercises, deep breathing, elastic stockings, early ambulation, monitoring dressings and drainage, wound care, adequate fluid intake, allow verbalization of feelings.*

5. **What are her likely psychosocial nursing diagnoses?**
   - *Anxiety related to cancer diagnosis, perceived loss of femininity, or disfigurement.*
   - *Body image disturbance related to altered fertility.*
   - *Knowledge deficit related to perioperative aspects of hysterectomy and self-care.*
   - *Grieving related to recent loss of spouse.*

6. **What are the discharge teaching needs for this client?**
   - *Resume activities slowly. Report signs/symptoms of infection (elevated temperature), DVT (redness, calf pain) or urinary problems (frequency, dysuria). Follow-up appointments. Suture/dressing care. May feel fatigued/weak for a few weeks. May experience emotional changes related to loss of ovarian hormones. Will have no further menstruation. Education relating to replacement hormones if prescribed and pain medications.*

CHAPTER 8

ANTIBIOTICS

Aminoglycoside prototype
gentamicin sulfate (Garamycin)

Pharmacodynamics--Inhibits protein synthesis and destroys susceptible organisms
Indications for use--Pseudomonas, escherichia coli, klebsiella, proteus, and staphylococcus infections. Endocarditis prophylaxis prior to surgery for clients with some heart disorders.
Adverse effects--Ototoxicity (hearing loss, tinnitus), vertigo, nephrotoxicity (oliguria and proteinuria), thrombocytopenia
Nursing considerations--Assess and monitor the client's hearing level. Teach the client about adverse effects and to notify his health care provider if they occur; tell him to increase fluid intake to 2 liters a day to prevent nephrotoxicity. Monitor peak/trough levels, BUN, creatinine.

Penicillin prototype
amoxicillin trihydrate (Amoxil)

Pharmacodynamics--Inhibits cell wall synthesis during bacterial multiplication and destroys susceptible bacteria such as staphylococcus, pseudomonas, meningitis, and gonorrhea
Indications for use--Infections by some gram-negative and gram-positive organisms. Endocarditis prophylaxis before dental surgery for clients with some heart disorders.
Adverse effects--Nausea, vomiting, diarrhea, allergic reactions, anemia
Nursing considerations--Assess the client's prior sensitivity to penicillins. Teach him to take with food to avoid GI upset, to take entire supply of drug to avoid developing drug-resistant strain, and to contact his health care provider if adverse effects develop (especially rash, fever, or chills) or if infection symptoms persist.

Cephalosporin prototype
cephalexin (Keflex)

Pharmacodynamics--Inhibits cell wall synthesis and promotes osmotic instability and destroys susceptible bacteria such as staphylococcus, pseudomonas, meningitis, and gonorrhea
Indications for use--Infections by some gram-negative and gram-positive organisms. Surgical prophylaxis for some clients.
Adverse effects--Rash, allergic reactions, nausea, vomiting, diarrhea
Nursing considerations--Assess prior sensitivity to penicillins and cephalosporins. Teach the client to take this drug with food to avoid GI upset and to take complete course of therapy to avoid developing resistance.

Macrolide prototype
azithromycin (Zithromax)

Pharmacodynamics--Binds to 50S subunit of bacterial ribosomes in susceptible organisms, inhibiting protein synthesis
Indications for use--Prophylaxis or treatment of infections caused by some gram-negative, gram-positive, and atypical organisms
Adverse effects--Nausea, vomiting, diarrhea, metallic taste (especially Biaxin), candidiasis, angioedema
Nursing considerations--Teach the client to take all of the prescribed dose. He should take it 1 hour before or 2 hours after meals because food decreases absorption.

Fluoroquinolon prototype
ciprofloxacin (Cipro)

Pharmacodynamics--Inhibits DNA synthesis, mainly by blocking DNA-Gyrase, which is necessary for bacterial DNA replication.
Indications for use--For treatment of infections caused by most gram-negative and some gram-positive bacteria
Adverse effects--Headache, vertigo, nausea, vomiting, diarrhea, crystalluria
Nursing considerations--Clients should be well-hydrated and avoid caffeine, excessive sunlight, tasks requiring alertness.

Sulfonamide prototype
co-trimoxazole (Bactrim)

Pharmacodynamics--Decreases bacterial folic acid synthesis, bacteriocidal
Indications for use--Urinary infections, chronic bronchitis, prophylaxis for pneumocystic disease, OM in clients allergic to penicillin
Adverse effects--Nausea, vomiting, diarrhea, toxic nephrosis, hemolytic and aplastic anemia, skin sensitivity, and pruritus
Nursing considerations--Assess the client for hypersensitivity. Teach him to increase fluid intake, to take all of the prescribed dose, to avoid prolonged exposure to sunlight, to report any signs of adverse reactions, and not to use birth-control pills.

ANTITUBERCULARS

Antitubercular prototype
isoniazid (Laniazid)

Pharmacodynamics--Acts against actively growing tubercle bacillus by interfering with lipid and DNA synthesis, thus inhibiting cell wall biosynthesis.

Indications for use--Pulmonary tuberculosis; some strains of mycobacterium bovis
Adverse effects--Peripheral neuropathy, nausea and vomiting, dry mouth, hepatitis, blood dyscrasia
Nursing considerations--Teach the client to take this drug exactly as prescribed and not to discontinue without prescriber's approval. Teach him to avoid alcohol, to take with food if GI irritation occurs, and to notify health care provider if symptoms of hepatitis develop. Monitor for peripheral paresthesia.

ANTIVIRALS

Antiviral prototype
acyclovir (Zovirax)

Pharmacodynamics--Interferes with DNA synthesis, inhibits viral multiplication, and destroys living viruses
Indications for use--Genital herpes and chicken pox
Adverse effects--Headache, tremors, confusion, nausea and vomiting, and skin rash, blood dyscrasia, acute renal failure
Nursing considerations--Teach the client that this drug controls herpes but does not cure it and will not prevent spread of infection to others. Recommend increased fluid intake to minimize dehydration from GI upset, and teach him about the symptoms of early herpes infection so drug therapy can be instituted.

ANTIFUNGALS

Antifungal prototype
nystatin (Mycostatin)

Pharmacodynamics--Binds to sterols in fungal cell membranes, altering permeability and allowing leakage of cell components
Indications for use--Local infections caused by candida
Adverse effects--Nausea, vomiting, local irritation, diarrhea
Nursing considerations--Shake suspension well; may use swish and swallow or swish and spit. Explain predisposing factors of vaginal infection, and advise the client to continue medication for at least 2 days after symptoms disappear.

ANTIHISTAMINES

Antihistamine prototype
diphenhydramine (Benadryl)

Pharmacodynamics--Competes with histamine for H_1-receptor sites on effector cells. Relieves allergy symptoms by preventing histamine-mediated

responses; also relieves motion sickness and cough; promotes sleep, and produces a calming effect.
Indications for use--Allergy symptoms, nasal stuffiness, motion sickness, non-productive cough, and sedation
Adverse effects--Nausea, dry mouth, drowsiness, palpitations, dysuria
Nursing considerations--Use cautiously in clients with angle-closure glaucoma, benign prostatic hyperplasia, asthma, and hypertension. Teach the client to take this drug with food or milk to avoid GI disturbances, to use ice chips or hard candy to relieve dry mouth, and to avoid activities that require being alert.

ANTINEOPLASTICS

Antineoplastic prototype
cyclophosphamide (Citizen)

Pharmacodynamics--Destroys specific types of cancer cells by interfering with RNA transcription; cell cycle-nonspecific
Indications for use--Various susceptible cancers, Hodgkin's disease, chronic lymphocytic leukemia, acute myelocytic leukemia
Adverse effects--Nausea and vomiting, stomatitis, hemorrhagic cystitis, thrombocytopenia, leukopenia, reversible alopecia
Nursing considerations--Prepare the client for impending alopecia; teach him that hair will regrow. Tell him not to take OTC medications; emphasize importance of increasing fluid intake to 3 liters a day to avoid hemorrhagic cystitis; teach him to watch for signs of infection and to notify health care provider if they occur. Both male and female clients taking drug should practice contraception while taking it and for 4 months following therapy because this drug is potentially teratogenic.

AUTONOMIC NERVOUS SYSTEM DRUGS

Parasympatholytic prototype
atropine sulfate

Pharmacodynamics--An anticholinergic that inhibits acetylcholine, blocking the effects of the vagus nerve, increasing the cardiac rate; decreases oral secretions and slows peristalsis
Indications for use--Bradycardia, antidote for anticholinesterase insecticide poisoning, preoperatively to decrease secretions and block vagus nerve reflexes
Adverse effects--Headache, restlessness, bradycardia after low dose, tachycardia after high dose, dry mouth, constipation, flushed face
Nursing considerations--Monitor the client for paradoxical bradycardia, initially; monitor cardiac clients for tachycardia. Teach the client to use hard candy to mitigate dry mouth. Do not give if client has glaucoma.

Parasympathomimetic prototype
neostigmine bromide (Prostigmin)

Pharmacodynamics--Stimulates muscle contractions by blocking destruction of acetylcholine
Indications for use--Myasthenia gravis diagnosis and treatment; postoperative abdominal distension; antidote for nondepolarizing neuromuscular blocking agents
Adverse effects--Nausea, vomiting, diarrhea, abdominal cramps, respiratory depression, bronchospasm, urinary frequency
Nursing considerations--Closely watch the client after each dose. Schedule dosing before muscle fatigue begins. Give oral dose with milk or food, and have atropine on hand in case adverse reaction occurs. Teach the client to wear medical identification device.

Sympathomimetic prototype
epinephrine (Adrenalin) [alpha and beta adrenergic]

Pharmacodynamics--Causes capillary arterial vasoconstriction, reduces nasal congestion, and reverses severe allergic reactions
Indications for use--Allergic reactions, nasal congestion, local bleeding, cardiac asystole, bronchospasm
Adverse effects--Tachycardia, nervousness, generalized feeling of excitation
Nursing considerations--Teach the client the correct use of metered-dose inhalers, about adverse effects; not to exceed prescribed dose; and to use only when indicated.. Monitor vital signs. Check peripheral vascular status with I.V. doses.

isoproterenol (Isuprel) [beta adrenergic]

Pharmacodynamics--Acting on beta$_2$-adrenergic receptors, relieves bronchospasm by relaxing bronchial smooth muscle; as a cardiac stimulant, acts on beta$_1$-receptors in the heart to relieve heart block and restore sinus rhythm following ventricular arrhythmias
Indications for use--To treat bronchial asthma and bronchospasm, heart block and some types of shock
Adverse effects--Headache, nervousness, cardiac palpitations, tachycardia, bronchial edema, diaphoresis, hyperglycemia
Nursing considerations--Teach the client how to use aerosol or sublingual form of drug and about overuse and the possibility of developing tolerance. Monitor ECG with I.V. doses, and do not exceed heart rate of 110/minute.

Sympatholytic prototype
prazosin (Minipress) [alpha antagonist]

Pharmacodynamics--Lowers blood pressure by blocking alpha adrenergic activity
Indications for use--Hypertension
Adverse effects--Orthostatic hypotension, dizziness, palpitations, blurred vision, impotence, nausea, dry mouth

Nursing considerations--Assess blood pressure regularly. Emphasize to the client that drug should not be stopped abruptly. Advise the client to minimize orthostatic hypotension by rising slowly and avoiding sudden position changes.

propranolol (Inderal) [beta antagonist]

Pharmacodynamics--Decreases the heart's oxygen demands by blocking catecholamine-induced increases in heart rate, blood pressure, and tone of myocardial contraction, thus relieving angina, reducing blood pressure, and aiding in limiting heart damage from an MI
Indications for use--Angina, various arrhythmias, hypertension, migraine headaches, mortality reduction post MI
Adverse effects--Nausea, general fatigue, lethargy, bradycardia, hypotension, heart failure, and intensification of AV block
Nursing considerations--Monitor the client's pulse rate. Teach the client to take his pulse before each dose and not to discontinue drug abruptly. Notify health care provider if pulse is very rapid or very slow. Contraindicated in clients with sinus bradycardia and heart block >first degree. Contraindicated in clients with bronchial asthma.

BLOOD COAGULATION MODIFIERS

Antiplatelet prototype
acetylsalicylic acid (Aspirin)

Pharmacodynamics--Blocks prostaglandin synthesis to produce analgesia, reduce clotting, and decrease inflammation; reduces fever by direct action on the hypothalamus
Indications for use--Mild to moderate pain, fever, inflammation, polyarthritic conditions, previous MI or unstable angina, stroke, reduced risk of heart attack or stroke (low dose)
Adverse effects--Reye's syndrome, nausea and vomiting, tinnitus, gastric upset, prolonged bleeding time, occult GI bleeding
Nursing considerations--Teach the client to take this drug with food, milk, or antacid, not to take any other over-the-counter (OTC) drugs without checking with his health care provider. If the client is on long-term therapy, check his salicylate serum level periodically. Do not administer to children or adolescents with chicken pox or flulike illness.

Anticoagulant prototype (injectable)
heparin sodium

Pharmacodynamics--Deactivates thrombin, preventing the conversion of fibrinogen to fibrin and thereby decreasing the blood's ability to clot
Indications for use--Deep vein thrombi, PE, MI, prevention of DVT, and emboli post-op (low dose)
Adverse effects--Hemorrhage, thrombocytopenia, hypersensitivity reactions, "white clot" syndrome
Nursing considerations--Begin bleeding precautions. Avoid I.M. injections. Teach the client to watch for signs of bleeding and to contact health care provider if bleeding occurs; emphasize that he should avoid OTC medications containing aspirin. Monitor partial thromboplastin time (PTT), anticoagulation values are 1½ to 2 times normal (control) values. Monitor platelet count.

Anticoagulant prototype (oral)
warfarin sodium (Coumadin)

Pharmacodynamics--Inhibits activation of vitamin K-dependent factors, decreasing the blood's clotting ability
Indications for use--MI, PE, valvular heart disease, chronic AF, DVT
Adverse effects--Hemorrhage, rash, fever, anorexia, nausea, vomiting, diarrhea
Nursing considerations--Monitor the client for bleeding. Teach him to avoid OTC medications containing salicylate and to use a soft toothbrush and an electric razor to avoid cutting the skin. He should avoid alcohol and limit intake of foods containing vitamin K because of their effect on anticoagulation. Advise client to wear a medical identification device. Monitor PT and INR (anticoagulation PT values are maintained at 1½ to 2 times normal range).

Low-molecular-weight heparin prototype
enoxaprin (Lovenox)

Pharmacodynamics--Accelerates formation of antithrombin IIIB-thrombin complex and deactivates thrombin, preventing conversion of fibrinogen to fibrin. Deactivates factor Xα, decreasing the blood's clotting ability
Indications for use--Prophylaxis of DVT and PE in orthopedic or abdominal surgery
Adverse effects--bleeding, thrombocytopenia, confusion, angioedema
Nursing considerations--Monitor for bleeding; monitor PT, INR, and platelet count. Monitor clients having epidural or spinal anesthesia for signs of neurologic impairment.

Thrombolytic prototype
streptokinase (Streptase)

Pharmacodynamics--Dissolves blood clots by activating plasminogen
Indications for use--Arterial and venous thrombi, pulmonary emboli, lysis of coronary artery thrombi following acute MI, occlusion of AV cannula
Adverse effects--Transient hypotension, bleeding, bronchospasm, flushed face, itching, reperfusion arrhythmias
Nursing considerations--Check for hypersensitivity reaction before administering. Draw blood for coagulation studies, hematocrit, platelet count and type and cross before beginning therapy. Monitor vital signs frequently. Use pressure dressings on all puncture sites. Handle the client carefully to avoid bruising. Avoid IM injections. Be aware that streptokinase must be administered within 6 hours of symptoms of onset for optimal effect.

CARDIOVASCULAR DRUGS

ACE inhibitor prototype
lisinopril (Zestril)

Pharmacodynamics--Prevents conversion of angiotensin I to angiotensin II, thereby suppressing renin-angiotensin-aldosterone system, lowering blood pressure, and improving renal function
Indications for use--Hypertension, cardiac failure
Adverse effects--Impotence, hypotension, angioedema, dry cough, anorexia, dizziness, fatigue, headache, blood dyscrasia
Nursing considerations--Teach the client to report any face, lips, or tongue swelling, shortness of breath, fever or sore throat. Explain that he may feel lightheaded; if he does, he should get up from sitting or lying slowly. Tell the client to call her health care provider if she gets pregnant.

Angiotensin II antagonist
losartan (Cozaar)

Pharmacodynamics--Inhibits binding of the vasoconstrictor angiotensin II to its receptor sites, found in many tissues, including vascular smooth muscle and adrenal glands
Indications for use--Hypertension
Adverse effects--Hypotension, dizziness, insomnia, nasal congestion
Nursing considerations--Not for use in pregnant women. Monitor blood pressure and renal function. Teach the client to avoid salt substitutes containing potassium.

Antiarrhythmic drugs

Atrial antiarrhythmia prototype
quinidine sulfate (Quinidex)

Pharmacodynamics--This class Ia antiarrhythmic restores normal sinus rhythm by a direct effect on the heart
Indications for use--Atrial flutter or fibrillation PACs and PVCs, paroxysmal SVT
Adverse effects--Dizziness, headache, fainting, acute asthma attack, diarrhea, nausea and vomiting, fever, tinnitus, hypotension
Nursing considerations--Emphasize that the client should take this drug with meals to avoid GI upset. Teach him about toxicity and when to report it. Monitor the client closely while he is on this drug, and emphasize the importance of keeping appointments with health care provider. Monitor pulse and serum quinidine levels.

Ventricular antiarrhythmic prototype
lidocaine (Xylocaine)

Pharmacodynamics--This Class 1b antiarrhythmic eliminates ventricular arrhythmias by direct action on the heart's Purkinje network to decrease depolarization, automaticity, and excitability
Indications for use--Ventricular arrhythmias, local and spinal anesthesia
Adverse effects--Double vision, confusion, tremors, depression, seizures, bradycardia, new or worsened arrhythmias
Nursing considerations--Monitor the client carefully for toxicity, and assess his vital signs regularly. Keep CPR equipment available. Give I.V. doses using a pump with client on continuous cardiac monitor. Discontinue infusion and notify cardiologist if toxicity occurs, arrhythmia worsens, or ECG shows widening QRS complex or prolonged PR interval

Antilipemic prototype
lovastatin (Mevacor)

Pharmacodynamics--Lowers low-density and total cholesterol by inhibiting the enzyme responsible for cholesterol synthesis
Indications for use--Reduction of elevated cholesterol levels and LDLs in clients with primary hypercholesterolemia
Adverse effects--Peripheral neuropathy, dizziness, heartburn, flatulence, muscle cramps, constipation, rhabdomyolisis
Nursing considerations--Teach the client to take with evening meals to enhance absorption. Store drug at room temperature and in a light-resistant

container. Warn the client to avoid alcohol because of potential for liver damage, and advise periodic eye exams (cataract formation).

Calcium channel blocker prototype
verapamil (Calan)

Pharmacodynamics--Relieves angina pectoris, decreases blood pressure, and restores sinus rhythm by inhibiting calcium ion transfer across cardiac and smooth muscle, thus decreasing myocardial contractility and oxygen demand. Also dilates coronary arteries and arterioles.
Indications for use--Angina pectoris, atrial fibrillation, hypertension, and various SVT arrhythmias
Adverse effects--Ventricular asystole, VF, transient hypotension, heart failure, constipation, dizziness, tiredness
Nursing considerations--Avoid use in nursing mothers. Teach the client to increase fluid and fiber intake to minimize constipation, to take drug with food, and to change position slowly to prevent dizziness. Monitor vital signs. Clients receiving I.V. drug form require continuous cardiac monitoring.

Cardiac glycoside prototype
digoxin (Lanoxin)

Pharmacodynamics--Improves myocardial contractions by promoting the transfer of calcium from extracellular to intracellular cytoplasm. Acts on CNS to enhance vagal tone, slowing conduction through SA and AV nodes and providing antiarrhythmic effect.
Indications for use--Congestive heart failure, atrial fibrillation and flutter, supraventricular tachycardia
Adverse effects--Arrhythmias, fatigue, muscle weakness, dizziness, blurred vision (especially yellow-green halos around images), anorexia, nausea and vomiting
Nursing considerations--Teach the client about adverse effects and to report any signs of toxicity immediately to health care provider. Monitor pulse rate; if sudden change to below 60 or above 120 bpm, consider withholding dose. Monitor serum potassium levels and take corrective action before hypokalemia occurs.

Vasodilator prototype
nitroglycerin (Nitrostat)

Pharmacodynamics--Relieves angina pectoris by reducing the heart's oxygen demands (reduces preload and, to a lesser extent, afterload). Also increases blood flow through collateral coronary arteries.

Indications for use--Prophylaxis for chronic angina pectoris attacks, treatment of acute attacks

Adverse effects--Postural hypotension, flushed face, tachycardia, throbbing headache, syncope, sublingual burning

Nursing considerations--Teach the client to apply transdermal patch to non-hairy parts of the body, to take sublingual tablet as soon as an attack begins, to keep these tablets away from heat and moisture, to check expiration date, and to avoid alcohol. Monitor vital signs.

CENTRAL NERVOUS SYSTEM DRUGS

Anticonvulsant prototype
phenytoin (Dilantin)

Pharmacodynamics--Stabilizes neuronal membranes and limits seizure activity by either increasing efflux or decreasing influx of sodium ions across cell membranes in motor cortex during generation of nerve impulses.

Indications for use--Generalized seizures, status epilepticus

Adverse effects--Hyperplasia of the gums, ataxia, slurred speech, nausea and vomiting, blood dyscrasia, rash, hirsutism, nystagmus, diplopia

Nursing considerations--Teach the client not to stop taking drug without his prescriber's permission; to perform good dental hygiene and to see a dentist regularly. Warn him that his urine may turn pink, red or brown, and tell him that if a rash develops, he should notify his health care provider. For I.V. administration, inject only into large veins or central venous catheter. Monitor CBC, serum calcium, and hepatic function periodically.

Antidepressant prototype
fluoxetine (Prozac)

Pharmacodynamics--Relieves depression and decreases obsessive-compulsive behavior, presumably by inhibiting CNS neuronal uptake of serotonin.

Indications for use--Depression, O/CDS

Adverse effects--Nervousness, nasal congestion, skin rash, itching, palpitations, hot flashes, dry mouth, weight loss, nausea, diarrhea, sexual dysfunction

Nursing considerations--Teach the client to take this drug in the morning to prevent insomnia, to avoid food high in tryptophan (meats, poultry, fish, liver, eggs, nuts, peanut butter), and to avoid hazardous activities requiring alertness until CNS effects are known. Do not give this drug to clients taking an MAOI. Order suicide precautions if necessary.

Antimanic prototype
lithium (Lithobid)

Pharmacodynamics--Prevents and controls manic behavior in bipolar disorders by altering neurochemical transmitters, possibly by interfering with ionic pump mechanisms in brain cells.

Indications for use--Bipolar disorder--manic episodes

Adverse effects--Arrhythmias, dry mouth, metallic taste, thirst, nausea and vomiting, increased urine output, skin rash, drowsiness, confusion, headache

Nursing considerations--Monitor blood glucose levels in clients with diabetes. Tell the client to increase his fluid intake up to 3,000 ml per day and to take this drug after meals to avoid GI upset. Teach him and his family about toxic effects (diarrhea, drowsiness, dizziness, ataxia); if they appear, he should withhold the next dose and call his health care provider immediately. Teach the client to wear a medical identification device, and warn him to expect a 3- or 4-week
delay before the drug is therapeutic. Monitor sodium intake, lithium blood levels, and urine specific gravity.

AntiParkinson agent prototype
carbidopa-levodopa (Sinemet)

Pharmacodynamics--Improves voluntary muscle movement by preventing depletion of dopamine and levodopa in the brain

Indications for use--Idiopathic Parkinson's disease and parkinsonian symptoms

Adverse effects--Jerking body movements, grimacing, postural hypotension, dry mouth, nausea and vomiting, diarrhea, cardiac irregularities, urinary frequency/retention, blood dyscrasia, hepatotoxity

Nursing considerations--Teach the client to rise slowly from sitting or lying position and to take the drug with food to minimize GI upset. Perform periodic blood glucose measurements if client is on long-term therapy. Teach him about adverse effects and to report them promptly to his health care provider.

Antipsychotic prototype
haloperidol (Haldol)

Pharmacodynamics--Reduces psychotic behavior by blocking postsynaptic dopamine receptors in the brain

Indications for use--Psychotic disorders; Tourette syndrome

Adverse effects--Extrapyramidal reactions (muscle spasms of tongue, face, neck and back, motor restlessness, and anxiety), tardive dyskinesia, seizures, dizziness, postural hypotension, dry mouth, urinary retention

Nursing considerations--Observe the client carefully for adverse effects. Teach the family about extrapyramidal adverse effects and to report them if they occur. Warn the client to avoid alcohol while on this drug, to take this drug exactly as prescribed, and not to discontinue it abruptly. Dilute oral concentration with water, orange juice, apple juice, or cola immediately prior to administration.

Barbiturate prototype
secobarbital (Seconal)

Pharmacodynamics--Promotes calmness and sleep by interfering with brain impulses from the thalamus to the cortex
Indications for use--Insomnia, preoperative sedation
Adverse effects--Hangover, drowsiness, respiratory depression, paradoxical excitement in the elderly
Nursing considerations--Be alert for clients hoarding drug for later suicide use. Teach the client about hangover adverse effect and that dreaming during sleep may be diminished; tell him to avoid alcohol. Use cautiously in the elderly because of greater sensitivity to the drug. If skin reaction occurs, discontinue the drug and notify health care provider (may precede potentially fatal reaction to therapy).

Benzodiazepine prototype
diazepam (Valium)

Pharmacodynamics--Depresses the CNS at the limbic and subcortical levels of the brain and relieves anxiety, promotes calmness, diminishes muscles spasms, suppresses spread of seizure activity produced by foci in the cortex, thalamus, and limbic structures
Indications for use--Preoperative sedation, anxiety, acute alcohol withdrawal, muscle spasms, seizure disorders, status epilepticus
Adverse effects--Depression, sleepiness, lethargy, bradycardia, urinary incontinence and retention
Nursing considerations--Teach the client to not do anything requiring alertness and dexterity until CNS effects of drug are known and to avoid alcohol. Warn the client and family about potential for dependency. Do not withdraw abruptly after long-term use.

Narcotic prototype
morphine sulfate (Duramorph)

Pharmacodynamics--Relieves pain by binding with opioid receptors in the brain, altering both perception of and emotional response to pain
Indications for use--Severe acute and chronic pain

Adverse effects--Respiratory depression, confusion, clouded mentation, sedation, hypotension, urinary retention, constipation, biliary tract spasms, physical dependence

Nursing considerations--Have narcotic antagonist available, and be prepared to institute resuscitation. Observe the client for respiratory depression before and after giving drug. Use with care in clients who are elderly, debilitated, or have head injuries. Morphine may worsen or mask gallbladder pain.

NSAID prototype
ibuprofen (Motrin)

Pharmacodynamics--Inhibits prostaglandin synthesis, producing anti-inflammatory, analgesic, and antipruritic effects

Indications for use--Prevention or treatment of pain, fever, or inflammation; dysmenorrhea, polyarthritis

Adverse effects--Nausea, gastritis, heartburn, bleeding from GI tract, urinary system, nose, etc., blood dyscrasia, bronchospasm, acute renal failure

Nursing considerations--Have the client take this drug with food to minimize GI upset. Unusual bleeding (urine, stool, etc.) must be reported immediately. Be aware that NSAIDs may mask signs and symptoms of infection.

Non-narcotic prototype
acetaminophen (Tylenol)

Pharmacodynamics--Blocks pain impulses in the brain and relieves mild pain and fever, probably by inhibiting prostaglandin or other substances that sensitive pain receptors. May relieve fever by action in the hypothalamic heat-regulating center.

Indications for use--Mild pain or fever

Adverse effects--Liver damage if large doses are taken or client consumes large quantities of alcohol; skin rash; hypoglycemia; blood dyscrasia

Nursing considerations--Monitor the client if taking zidovudine carefully (drug may cause bone marrow suppression). Teach him that this drug should be used for a short time only and to avoid alcohol because of increased risk of hepatic damage. Health care provider should be contacted if pain does not subside.

RENAL SYSTEM DRUGS

Loop diuretic prototype
furosemide (Lasix)

Pharmacodynamics--Stimulates water excretion by inhibiting NA+ and Cl⁻ reabsorption at the proximal and distal tubules and the ascending loop of Henle
Indications for use--Pulmonary and peripheral edema, hypertension
Adverse effects--Blood dyscrasia, orthostatic hypotension, polyuria, diarrhea, hypokalemia and dehydration; transitory deafness with rapid I.V. injection
Nursing considerations--Monitor the client's weight daily. Assess breath sounds, vital signs, and I&O. Teach the client to change position slowly to avoid postural hypotension, to watch for signs of hypokalemia, and about photosensitivity concerns. Advise client to report signs of toxicity immediately. Take his blood pressure and check potassium level before giving I.V.

Osmotic diuretic prototype
mannitol (Osmitrol)

Pharmacodynamics--Reduces intracranial and intraoptic pressure by elevating plasma osmolality, resulting in enhanced movement of intracellular fluid into vascular space; promotes water excretion by preventing water reabsorption in the kidneys
Indications for use--Test for suspected kidney disease, increased intracranial or intraocular pressure, edema from cardiac or kidney failure.
Adverse effects--Vascular overload leading to heart failure and pulmonary edema, diarrhea, blurred vision, urinary retention, thirst, fluid and electrolyte imbalance.
Nursing considerations--Monitor the client's vital signs, including central venous pressure (CVP), hourly. Monitor I&O daily. Warn the client that he will be thirsty but should not drink more than amount prescribed). Tell the client to report any chest pain to his health care provider. Assess weight, renal function, fluid balance, and serum and urine sodium and potassium.

Potassium-sparing diuretic prototype
spironolactone (Aldactone)

Pharmacodynamics--Stimulates water and sodium excretion but inhibits potassium excretion by antagonizing aldosterone effect in the distal tubules.

Indications for use--Edema, hypertension, hyperaldosteronism, congestive heart failure

Adverse effects--Increased potassium levels, dehydration, loss of appetite, nausea and vomiting, diarrhea, cramping, headache, ataxia

Nursing considerations--Monitor serum electrolytes, I&O, weight, and blood pressure. Teach the client not to eat of lot of potassium-containing foods like bananas and to take this drug with meals to avoid GI upset.

Thiazide diuretic prototype
hydrochlorothiazide (Hydrodiuril)

Pharmacodynamics--Inhibits reabsorption of sodium and chloride in renal distal tubules

Indications for use--Hypertension, mild edema

Adverse effects--Rash, hypercalcemia, dehydration, hypotension, renal failure

Nursing considerations--Not for use in pregnant women. Advise the client to take this drug in the morning to prevent nocturia, and teach him the signs of hypokalemia. Monitor fluid and electrolytes, creatinine, BUN, I&O, and blood pressure.

Uricosuric prototype
allopurinol (Zyloprim)

Pharmacodynamics--Reduces uric acid production by inhibiting biochemical reactions preceding its formation, thus relieving symptoms of gout

Indications for use--Gout, hyperuricemia

Adverse effects--Blood dyscrasia, skin rash, itching, abdominal pain, diarrhea, hepatitis, paresthesias, taste loss or perversion, GI upset, drowsiness

Nursing considerations--Teach the client to increase his fluid intake, to take this drug with meals to avoid GI upset, to avoid alcohol, to stop taking this drug if rash or other skin eruptions occur. Monitor serum uric acid levels to evaluate response. Monitor CBC and hepatic and renal function at start of therapy and periodically.

RESPIRATORY SYSTEM DRUGS

Bronchodilator prototype
theophylline (Theo-dur)

Pharmacodynamics--Improves breathing by relaxing smooth muscle tissue in the bronchi and pulmonary vessels
Indications for use--Acute and chronic bronchospasm
Adverse effects--Dizziness, restlessness, nausea and vomiting, tachycardia, skin itching, palpations, tachycardia, tachypnea
Nursing considerations--Monitor the client's vital signs. Tell the client not to chew a sustained-released capsule and to take with full glass of water; make sure he knows to take drug as prescribed and not to overuse it. Have the client check with his health care provider before taking any OTC medication. Tell him to take this drug in morning to avoid insomnia, and warn him that smoking increases elimination of theophylline, increasing dosage requirements. Monitor serum theophylline levels to avoid toxicity.

Mucolytic prototype
acetylcysteine (Mucomyst)

Pharmacodynamics--Thins and reduces viscosity of tenacious respiratory secretions; antagonizes toxic effects of acetaminophen by restoring liver stores of glutathione
Indications for use--Pneumonia, CF, acetaminophen overdose
Adverse effects--Bronchospasm, nausea and vomiting, rhinorrhea, tachycardia
Nursing considerations--Assess respiratory secretions before administering drug, and be alert for bronchospasm. Have the client clear his airway by coughing before using nebulizer form of drug. Effective treatment for acetaminophen overdose to begin within 24 hours after ingestion; begin treatment immediately after drug is prescribed. Warn the client that this drug has a very unpleasant odor.

Leukotriene inhibitor prototype
montelukast (Singulair)

Pharmacodynamics--Inhibits the binding of inflammatory leukotrienes to receptors in lungs, reducing bronchoconstriction caused by antigen challenge
Indications for use--Preventing asthma symptoms
Adverse effects--Headache, nausea, diarrhea
Nursing considerations--Teach the client to take drug daily, even if he is asymptomatic, and to notify his health care provider if his symptoms worsen. Not for acute asthma attacks or COPD.

OPHTHALMIC DRUGS

Miotic prototype
pilocarpine (Salagen)

Pharmacodynamics--This cholinergic causes pupillary contraction when topically applied to the eye and increases secretions of the exocrine glands (sweat, lacrimal, gastric, pancreatic, and intestinal glands)
Indications for use--Primary open angle glaucoma, hyposalivary disorders
Adverse effects--Blurred vision, conjunctival irritation, transient stinging and burning, brow pain, excessive sweating, headache, rhinitis, GI upset
Nursing considerations--Advise the client not to drive or use complicated equipment because of visual disturbances. He should increase fluid intake to compensate for sweating and prevent dehydration. Warn client about urinary frequency.

GASTROINTESTINAL SYSTEM DRUGS

Antacid prototype
aluminum hydroxide (Amphojel)

Pharmacodynamics--Diminishes gastric upset by reducing gastric acid; binds with phosphate in GI tract and elevating gastric pH
Indications for use--Gastric distress from hyperacidity, control of **hyperphoshatemia** in clients with renal failure
Adverse effects--Constipation, loss of appetite, intestinal obstruction
Nursing considerations--Avoid giving any other oral medications for 2 hours after giving antacid. Explain to the client that drug may color his stool white, and teach him techniques to reduce constipation.

Antidiarrheal prototype
diphenoxylate (Lomotil)

Pharmacodynamics--Inhibits intestinal motility and diminishes intestinal secretions
Indications for use--Diarrhea
Adverse effects--Paralytic ileus, dry mouth, abdominal discomfort or distention, urinary retention, dizziness, skin rash, respiratory depression, angioedema
Nursing considerations--Caution the client about long-term use over 2 days and about driving until effects of drug are known. Observe client for electrolyte disturbances. Be advised that drug is not indicated for treatment of antibiotic-induced diarrhea.

Antinausea/Antiemetic prototype
prochlorperazine (Compazine)

Pharmacodynamics--Acts on chemoreceptor trigger zone to decrease nausea and vomiting by depressing the vomiting center
Indications for use--Preoperative control of nausea, control of severe vomiting
Adverse effects--Orthostatic hypotension, blurred vision, dry mouth, constipation, urine retention, extrapyramidal adverse effects
Nursing considerations--Do not administer within 2 hours of giving an antacid. Teach the client to rise slowly to avoid postural hypotension, and to mix oral solution with juice, milk, or pudding. I.V. infusion should be administered slowly (not to exceed 5 mg/minute).

H_2-receptor antagonist prototype
cimetidine (Tagamet)

Pharmacodynamics--Reduces gastric irritation by inhibiting histamine action at receptor sites of parital cells, decreasing gastric acid secretion
Indications for use--Heartburn, duodenal ulcer, gastroesophageal reflux disease (GERD), prevention of stress ulcers in critically ill clients.
Adverse effects--Blood dyscrasias, diarrhea, itching, skin rash, headache
Nursing considerations--Teach the client to take this drug with meals or at bedtime if taken only once daily and not to take this drug within 2 hours of taking an antacid. Encourage the client to stop smoking because it increases gastric acid secretion. Warn client to call his health care provider if his stools become unusually dark or if he develops a skin rash.

Proton pump inhibitor prototype
omeprazole (Prilosec)

Pharmacodynamics--Blocks the formation of gastric acid by inhibiting the activity of the acid (proton) pump and binding to hydrogen/potassium adenosine triphosphatase located at the secretory surface of gastric parietal cells
Indications for use--Gastric or duodenal ulcer, GERD
Adverse effects--Headache, dizziness, diarrhea, nausea and vomiting, constipation, flatulence
Nursing considerations--Best if the capsule is swallowed whole, although it can be opened and the contents administered through a large-bore feeding tube. This drug should be taken before meals.

Stool-softener prototype
docusate sodium (Colace)

Pharmacodynamics--Softens stool by reducing surface tension of intestinal fluids and promoting incorporation of additional liquids into stools, forming a softer mass
Indications for use--Any need to soften the stool
Adverse effects--Abdominal cramps, throat irritation, bitter taste, diarrhea
Nursing considerations--Teach the client foods to eat that provide dietary bulk. Tell him to stop taking this drug if abdominal cramps occur, and teach him to mix the liquid form in milk, juice, or soda to mask the bitter taste.

ENDOCRINE SYSTEM DRUGS
Antidiabetics

Insulin prototype
regular insulin (Humulin)

Pharmacodynamics--Increases glucose transport across muscle and fat cell membranes to reduce blood glucose levels
Indications for use--DM
Adverse effects--Itching, skin rash, swelling at the injection site, lipoatrophy hypoglycemia
Nursing considerations--Teach the client about DM and the need to exercise, to eat a proper diet, and to take insulin as prescribed. Teach him how to monitor his blood glucose levels; review the signs of hypoglycemia and what to do if it occurs. Note that regular insulin is the only insulin that can be given I.V. Client should wear a medic alert device at all times.

Sulfonylurea prototype
tolbutamide (Orinase)

Pharmacodynamics--Stimulates release of insulin from the pancreatic cells and reduces glucose output by liver; extrapancreatic effect is an increased peripheral sensitivity to insulin
Indications for use--Adult onset (type 2) DM
Adverse effects--Skin rash, photosensitivity, GI upset, anemia, hypoglycemia, blood dyscrasias, blurred vision, hypoglycemia
Nursing considerations--Watch for adverse effects. Monitor the client's blood glucose levels. Teach the client to take drug as ordered and to not change brands without asking his health care provider; teach him about DM and steps to maintain good blood glucose control. Hypoglycemia induced by tolbutamide may persist for 24 to 48 hours. Advise the client that during periods of stress (infection, surgery, trauma), he may need insulin therapy.

Biguanide prototype
metformin (Glucophage)

Pharmacodynamics--Slows glucose production in the liver and absorption in the intestines; increases peripheral glucose uptake and utilization
Indications for use--Adult onset (type 2) DM
Adverse effects--Lactic acidosis, GI upset, weight loss, metallic taste in the mouth, vitamin B_{12} deficiency
Nursing considerations--Monitor the client's blood glucose level. Teach the client about DM and self-monitoring techniques. Watch for signs of metabolic acidosis. Teach client signs of acidosis and tell him to stop the drug if they appear and call his health care provider. Administer with meals. Arrange for periodic testing of vitamin B_{12} level. Clients should wear medic alert device at all times.

Thiazolidinedione prototype
troglitazone (Rezulin)

Pharmacodynamics--Inhibits hepatic glucose production and improves cell response to insulin
Indications for use--Adjunct to diet and insulin therapy in clients with type 2 DM whose hyperglycemia is inadequately controlled with insulin therapy over 30 units per day
Adverse effects--Headache, UTI, hepatotoxicity
Nursing considerations--Teach the client about the disease and how to manage for good blood glucose control. Monitor the client's blood glucose level frequently until appropriate level is established. Emphasize that this drug should be taken with meals. Monitor liver enzymes at start of therapy and every 6 months. Clients should wear medic alert device at all times.

Glucocorticoids

Drug prototype
prednisone (Deltasone)

Pharmacodynamics--Decreases inflammation and suppresses immune response; stimulates bone marrow; influences protein, fat and carbohydrate metabolism
Indications for use--Severe inflammatory response, chronic respiratory disorders, autoimmune disorders, immunosuppression
Adverse effects--Adrenal insufficiency with increased stress or abrupt withdrawal of long-term therapy, gastric ulcer, hypertension, skin eruptions, hyperglycemia, euphoria, insomnia, cushingoid state, osteoporosis, muscle weakness
Nursing considerations--Be sure that the drug is not confused with

prednisolone. Teach the client to not stop taking drug without his health care provider's consent, and warn him to report any weight loss, swelling in the extremities, or signs of adrenal insufficiency (weakness, fatigue, fever, joint pain). Teach him about body image changes (i.e., moon face) after long-term use. Give as once-daily dose in the morning for better results and less toxicity; give with food to decrease GI irritation. Weigh daily and report sudden increases. When therapy is to end, reduce dosage gradually to prevent adrenal insufficiency.

Thyroid drugs

Antithyroid prototype
propylthiouracil (PTU)

Pharmacodynamics--Inhibits oxidation of iodine in the thyroid, blocking iodine's ability to combine with tyrosine to form T4; may prevent coupling of monoiodotyrosine and diiodotyrosine to form T4 and T3; lowers thyroid hormone level
Indications for use--Hyperthyroidism, thyrotoxic crisis
Adverse effects--Liver toxicity, blood dyscrasias, nausea and vomiting, visual disturbances, headache, drowsiness, vertigo, loss of taste
Nursing considerations--Observe the client for signs of hypothyroidism (edema, mental depression, edema). Teach him to report any skin rash to his health care provider, and advise him to take this drug with meals to avoid GI upset.

Thyroid-replacement prototype
levothyroxine (Synthroid)

Pharmacodynamics--Raises thyroid hormone levels and stimulates general metabolism by accelerating the rate of cellular oxidation
Indications for use--Myxedema, cretinism, hypothyroidism
Adverse effects--Tremors, feelings of excitability, tachycardia, hypertension, changes in menstruation, insomnia, palpitations, diarrhea, heat intolerance
Nursing considerations--Emphasize need for strict compliance to maintain desired hormone level. Teach the client to take this drug in morning to avoid insomnia and to report any signs of cardiac distress (sweating, dyspnea, palpitations). Be aware that clients requiring ^{131}I uptake studies must discontinue the drug 4 weeks prior to test.

REPRODUCTIVE SYSTEM DRUGS

Estrogen prototype
conjugated estrogen (Premarin)

Pharmacodynamics--Improves the synthesis of DNA, RNA, and protein in responsive tissues; reduces release of follicle-stimulating hormone and leutinizing hormone from the pituitary gland
Indications for use--Uterine bleeding, breast cancer, symptoms of menopause, inoperable prostate cancer, osteoporosis
Adverse effects--Embolism, thrombophlebitis, nausea, breast enlargement and tenderness, vision changes, increased risk of endometrial cancer
Nursing considerations--Warn the client about adverse effects and tell her to report any signs of thromboembolitic disease. Do careful physical and history before administering drug. Teach the client to do periodic breast examination. Recommend yearly Pap test, thorough physical exam, serum lipid monitoring, and liver functions as appropriate.

Oxytocic prototype
oxytocin (Pitocin)

Pharmacodynamics--Stimulates uterine and mammary gland smooth muscle
Indications for use--Induce labor, stop uterine bleeding after placenta expulsion, incomplete abortion
Adverse effects--Maternal: hypertension, arrhythmias, generalized seizures, nausea and vomiting, uterine rupture; fetal: bradycardia, anoxia, brain damage
Nursing considerations--Assess the client's uterine contractions. Assess adequacy of pelvic measurements and fetal lie; assess fetal status. Use only as an I.V. infusion, not bolus dose. Monitor the client's fluid I&O.

Progestin prototype
progesterone (Gesterol 50)

Pharmacodynamics--Inhibits pituitary gonadotropin gland secretion, stopping ovulation; forms thick cervical mucus
Indications for use--Dysfunctional uterine bleeding, amenorrhea, contraception
Adverse effects--Pulmonary embolus, abdominal cramps, breast tenderness
Nursing considerations--Monitor injection sites for irritation if giving drug I.M. As required by law, have the client read package insert prior to giving first dose, then document that she has read and understood the insert. Tell her to stop taking this drug if migraine occurs or vision changes and to call her health care provider immediately. Recommend yearly Pap test.